HRT:
The Answers

HRT:
The Answers

*A Concise Guide for Solving
the Hormone Replacement
Therapy Puzzle*

Pamela Wartian Smith, M.D., MPH

Healthy Living Books, Inc.
TRAVERSE CITY, MICHIGAN

Although the author and publisher have made every effort to ensure the accuracy and completeness of information contained in this book, we assume no responsibility for errors, inaccuracies, omissions, or any inconsistency herein. Any slights of people, places, or organizations are unintentional.

First printing 2003

ISBN 0-9729767-3-6
LCCN 2003103384

ATTENTION CORPORATIONS, UNIVERSITIES, COLLEGES, AND PROFESSIONAL ORGANIZATIONS: Quantity discounts are available on bulk purchases of this book for educational, gift purposes, or as premiums for increasing magazine subscriptions or renewals. Special books or book excerpts can also be created to fit specific needs. For information, please contact Healthy Living Books, Inc., 575 S. Long Lake Road, Traverse City, MI 49684, ph 231-943-4577.

Dedication

To my daughters, Autumn, Hollie and Caitlin, who are now just learning the importance of hormones.

To my husband Christopher, whose patience with me as I traveled along my own hormonal "journey" has been nothing short of wonderful.

Thanks

Thank you to the librarians at St. Joseph Mercy Hospital in Ann Arbor, Michigan. Without their help, this book would never have been written.

Disclaimer

The information contained in this book is designed for information and education only and is not intended to prescribe treatment.

In order to accommodate new medical research as it was unfolding, the references in the body of the text are not sequentially numbered.

To see a board-certified physician in your area who specializes in customized, prescription hormone replacement, contact the American Academy of Anti-Aging Physicans: 1-773-528-4333 or visit them on the web at: www.worldhealth.net.

Table of Contents

Foreword ● *ix*

Introduction ● *1*

Hormone Replacement Therapy (HRT) ● *3*

Should You Take HRT? ● *7*

Estrogen ● *10*

Synthetic Estrogen ● *14*

Natural Estrogens ● *17*

Estrogen Metabolism ● *21*

Estrogen and Your Brain ● *26*

Estrogen Receptor Modulators ● *28*

Progesterone ● *29*

Estrogen/Progesterone Ratio ● *35*

Testosterone ● *36*

DHEA ● *40*

Cortisol ● *42*

Insulin and Your Sex Hormones ● *45*

Thyroid Hormone ● *46*

Melatonin ● *52*

Pregnenolone ● *54*

Prolactin ● *55*

Detoxification ● *57*

Osteoporosis ● *63*

Secondary Risk Factors for Heart Disease ● *70*

Nutrition ● *74*

Hormones and Your Skin ● *76*

Birth Control Pills ● *78*

Weight Gain in Menopause ● *79*

Surgical Menopause ● *81*

Herbal Therapies for Menopause ● *82*

Salivary Testing ● *83*

Compounded Hormones ● *84*

Conclusion ● *85*

Appendix I: Compounding Pharmacies ● *87*

Appendix II: Laboratories ● *89*

Appendix III: Supplements ● *90*

Appendix IV: Companies that Use
Pharmaceutical Grade Supplements ● *91*

References and Notes ● *92*

Foreword

With the completion of the Genome Project, it is now possible to individualize or customize treatment plans for each person. How you metabolize medication, or what you need are very different from your mother, your sister, or your friend.

Much of this book is written in concise, bullet style format, as opposed to long literary prose. It was designed as such for today's busy woman who does not want to wade through extraneous sentence structure. You can, therefore, see the important points at a moment's glance. Consequently, many of the lengthy scientific explanations are not present in the body of this text.

For those of you who want a further explanation of the principles contained in this book, please avail yourself of the numerous citations from the medical journals in the reference section of this manuscript.

It is my hope that this book will serve as a reference for all peri-menopausal and menopausal women so that we can each receive the individualized care that we all deserve.

In good health,

Pamela W. Smith, M.D., MPH

"All of the hormones in your body are designed to work together. This is God's plan. Therefore, if one is altered, or deficient, it will affect the actions of all of the other hormones in your body."

—PAMELA W. SMITH, M.D., MPH

Introduction

This book was written to herald a new age in medicine. With the completion of the Genome Project, we now have the medical capability to develop and customize a treatment plan for each patient. Gone will be the days of protocols.

The subsequent pages of this text will look at the intricate web of your body's hormonal system. The first few chapters look at your sex hormones: estrogen, progesterone, testosterone, DHEA, and cortisol. Subsequent chapters discuss other hormones: thyroid, insulin, melatonin, prolactin, and pregnenolone, all of which interface with your sex hormones. Other chapters will deal with the metabolism (breakdown) and detoxification of estrogen in your body. Later chapters will look at the prevention and treatment of osteoporosis and heart disease in women, as well as, weight gain during menopause, and hormones and your skin.

The correct levels of all of your hormones are needed for you to achieve optimal health.

"It is impossible to achieve optimum health without a properly functioning hormonal system."

—DAVID BROWNSTEIN, M.D.,
The Miracle of Natural Hormones

Hormone Replacement Therapy (HRT)

Every day in the United States 3,500 women enter menopause.[113] Menopause is defined as no menstrual cycle for 12 months. Symptoms, however, can begin as long as fifteen years prior to menopause.

Symptoms of menopause:

- Hot flashes
- Night sweats
- Vaginal dryness
- Vaginal odor
- Mood swings
- Irritability
- Insomnia
- Depression
- Loss of sexual interest
- Hair growth on face
- Painful intercourse
- Panic attacks
- Weird dreams
- Urinary tract infections
- Vaginal itching
- Lower back pain
- Bloating
- Flatulence (gas)
- Indigestion
- Osteoporosis
- Aching ankles, knees, wrists, shoulders, heels
- Hair loss
- Frequent urination
- Snoring
- Sore breasts
- Palpitations
- Varicose veins
- Urinary leakage
- Dizzy spells
- Panic attacks
- Skin feeling crawly
- Migraine headaches
- Memory lapses

The normal age to go through menopause ranges from 35 to 55. Therefore, you may easily live one half of your life without a menstrual cycle.

Until recently, the only hormonal therapy available in this country has been synthetic hormone replacement.

The government sponsored Women's Health Initiative Program halted its study on estrogen plus progestin, (synthetic progesterone, Prempro), on July 9, 2002. This was three years early because of an increased risk of breast cancer in women taking these hormones.[318] Analysis of the study also revealed that heart attack risk began increasing in the progestin group early in the study which was conducted on 16,000 women who had not had a hysterectomy. Participants in the study were either given Prempro or a placebo.

The study revealed the following results:[318]

- The stroke rate was 41% higher in women taking Prempro.
- Women on Prempro had double the rate of blood clots.
- Women on Prempro had an increase in breast cancer of 26%.
- Women on Prempro had a 22% increase in heart disease.
- Women on Prempro had a 37% decrease in colorectal cancer.
- Women on Prempro had a decrease in fracture rate of the hip of 33%.
- Women on Prempro had a decrease in total fracture rate of 24%.

The trial is continuing for women taking estrogen without progestin (synthetic progesterone).

Additional studies, such as the Heart and Estrogen/Progestin Replacement Study Follow-up (HERS II), agree with the findings of the Women's Health Initiative Trial. Results also showed an increase in cardiovascular risk in women taking synthetic progesterone.[320] Likewise, several other studies have shown recently that progestins (synthetic progesterone) have an unfavorable effect on cholesterol levels and may promote cardiovascular disease.[319]

Synthetic HRT has also been shown to have other problems:

- It is estimated that one-half of women quit taking their synthetic hormone replacement therapy after one year because they are unable to tolerate the side effects.[7]

- Synthetic hormones waste energy by giving incomplete messages to cells which then fail to produce a balanced hormonal response.[397]

The results of the Women's Health Initiative Study brought to the forefront why synthetic hormonal therapy will quickly become a treatment of the past. *In the following pages you will discover the answer to HRT: customized natural hormone replacement that is a prescription.*

"Today's truth is this: There is no magic hormone or combination of hormones that can be indiscriminately used by all women. Each woman is an individual and hormonal balance must be the ultimate goal for all women."

—JOSEPH COLLINS, N.D.,
What's Your Menopause Type

Should You Take HRT?

The results of the Women's Health Initiative Study highlights the problems associated with "one-size fits all" medicine. What is needed is to more carefully evaluate your own *unique* set of environmental, genetic, and physiological risk factors.

What is natural hormone replacement? Natural hormone replacement means using hormones that are biologically identical to what your body makes. In other words, the hormones are the same chemical structure as the ones that your body made before menopause.

Customized natural hormonal therapy is the only way to replace hormones safely. One size does not fit all. Now there is a more effective way. Studies have shown that women who use hormone replacement live longer than those who do not.[418]

Your hormone response is as unique to you as your fingerprints. How you respond to HRT is related to your genetic profile, stress level, condition of your health, your environment, nutritional supplementation, and what you are eating.

Hormone replacement should not be considered without a thorough understanding of how all of your body's hormones interact with each other. For example, insulin resistance and hyperinsulinemia (uncontrolled blood sugar) influence the synthesis of testosterone and the metabolism of DHEA in women.[89] Consequently, insulin resistance increases testosterone production and depletes DHEA in the body. This occurs because the increase in insulin elevates the activity of an enzyme, 17, 20

7

lyase, which converts more DHEA to cortisol and testosterone. This encourages obesity.

To take this concept one step further, a study done at the University of Toronto revealed a 283% increase in the risk of breast cancer if insulin levels are elevated.[304] There are insulin receptors on breast cells. Cancer cells also have insulin receptors. Insulin attaches to the receptor and turns it on which increases the growth of cancer cells. *Therefore, if your blood sugar is high you may be increasing your risk of breast cancer.*

There are five reasons you should consider natural hormone replacement therapy:
- Relief of symptoms
- Prevention of memory loss
- Heart health
- Bone production (prevention of osteoporosis)
- Growth and repair

Hormones that regulate growth and repair:
- Insulin
- Growth hormone
- Testosterone
- Estrogens
- DHEA

The ratio between all of your hormones is also important for optimal health.

If you have a low progesterone to estrogen ratio you may experience any of the following:[166]
- Infertility
- Abnormal bleeding in peri and postmenopause
- Increased risk of breast cancer
- Increased risk of uterine cancer

***If your progesterone to estrogen ratio is too* high,
you may have problems with the following:[167]**

- Insulin resistance/diabetes
- Depression
- Fatigue
- Decrease in sexual interest

Subsequent chapters will look at the ratios of your hormones in a more in-depth manner.

Is there an increased risk of cancer if you take hormone replacement therapy? 90% of postmenopausal women who develop breast cancer have never taken any kind of hormone replacement therapy [419] In the following chapters you will learn how prescription natural hormonal therapy may actually *decrease* your risk of developing cancer.

When you stop taking hormone replacement therapy you lose the benefits that hormones provide almost immediately.

Estrogen

Estrogen has 400 crucial functions in your body, including the following:[195, 196, 549, 40, 61]

- Stimulates the production of choline acetyltransferase, an enzyme, which prevents Alzheimer's disease[416, 486, 392, 393, 349]
- Increases your metabolic rate
- Improves insulin sensitivity[493, 201, 503, 504]
- Regulates body temperature
- Helps prevent muscle damage[214]
- Helps maintain muscle[213, 229]
- Helps you sleep deeply[232]
- Reduces your risk of cataracts[54]
- Helps maintain the elasticity of your arteries[52]
- Dilates your small arteries[52, 545]
- Increases blood flow[52, 405, 311]
- Inhibits platelet stickiness[52]
- Decreases the accumulation of plaque on your arteries[52]
- Enhances magnesium uptake and utilization[473]
- Maintains the amount of collagen in your skin
- Decreases blood pressure[492]
- Decreases LDL (bad cholesterol) and prevents its oxidation[487, 547]
- Helps maintain your memory[482, 483, 484, 409, 410, 411, 412]
- Increases reasoning and new ideas[485, 582]
- Helps with fine motor skills[485, 582]

- Increases the water content of your skin and is responsible for its thickness and softness[481]
- Enhances the production of nerve-growth factor[317]
- Increases HDL (good cholesterol) by 10 to 15%[543]
- Reduces the overall risk of heart disease by 40 to 50%[543]
- Decreases lipoprotein A (a risk factor for heart disease)[544]
- Acts as a natural calcium channel blocker to keep your arteries open[546]
- Enhances energy[210]
- Improves your mood[201]
- Increases concentration[201]
- Maintains bone density[201, 495]
- Increases sexual interest[201]
- Reduces homocysteine (a risk factor for heart disease)[116, 117]
- Decreases wrinkles[100]
- Protects against macular degeneration[100]
- Decreases your risk of colon cancer[100]
- Helps prevent tooth loss[100]
- Aids in the formation of neurotransmitters in your brain such as serotonin which decreases depression, irritability, anxiety, and pain sensitivity[202, 203, 263]

Your body has receptor sites for estrogen everywhere: in your brain, muscles, bone, bladder, gut, uterus, ovaries, vagina, breast, eyes, heart, lungs, and blood vessels.

The following are symptoms of decreased estrogen:
- Thinner skin
- More wrinkles/aging skin
- Decrease in breast size
- Stress incontinence
- Oily skin
- Acne
- Decreased sex drive
- Decreased dexterity
- Increase in insulin resistance and possible diabetes

- Vaginal dryness
- Decreased memory
- Osteoporosis
- Urinary tract infections
- Increased cholesterol

Other interesting facts:

- Estrogen levels are lower in women who smoke. This may be why women who smoke have more menopausal symptoms than women who do not smoke.[152]

- Stress suppresses estrogen function.[262]

- Hot flashes may be due to the fluctuating levels of estrogen rather than a true decrease in estrogen.[62]

- Eating high fat foods can increase your liver recirculation of your estrogens. This keeps estrogen circulating in your body and may predispose you to breast cancer.[424]

- A high fat diet increases estradiol (E2, see the chapter on natural estrogen) production by 30%.[295]

- Low fat diets decrease free estrogen (the amount available for usage by your body).[296]

- Omega-3-fatty acids can decrease the effect of estrogen.[298]

- Estrogen can be reabsorbed back into your blood stream again. This can happen with leaky gut syndrome or when there is not enough fiber to bind estrogen and propel it through your bowel.

- Researchers have concluded that estrogen use would decrease the rate of heart disease by almost 50%.[48, 378]

You can have too much estrogen in your body. Dr. John Lee coined the phrase "estrogen dominance" to describe symptoms of estrogen excess.[162]

Symptoms of estrogen excess:[163, 140]

- Cervical dysplasia
- Decreased sexual interest
- Depression with anxiety or agitation
- Increased risk of cancer of the uterus
- Weight gain (especially abdomen, hips, thighs)
- Water retention
- Headaches
- Poor sleep
- Panic attacks
- Swollen breasts
- Heavy periods
- Increased risk of breast cancer
- Increased risk of auto-immune diseases
- Hypothyroidism (increases the binding of thyroid hormone)[142]
- Fatigue
- Fibrocystic breasts
- Irritability
- Mood swings
- Uterine fibroids
- Bloating

Estrogen dominance can result from the over production of estrogen or from an imbalance of progesterone to estrogen. The symptoms of estrogen excess may also be the result of the transformation of estrogens, rather than with the absolute amount of estrogen in your system. (See the chapter on estrogen metabolism.)

Causes of excess estrogen in your body:[63]

- Taking too much estrogen
- Impaired elimination of estrogen
- Lack of exercise
- Diet low in grains and fiber
- Environmental estrogens (See the chapter on estrogen metabolism.)
- Elevation of 16-hydroxyestrone metabolism (See the chapter on estrogen metabolism.)

Synthetic Estrogen

The most commonly prescribed hormone replacement in the U.S. is Premarin. Premarin is a mixture of:

- Estrone (as sodium estrone sulfate)
- Sodium equilin sulfate
- Concomitant components as:
  - −17 alpha-dihydroequilin
  - −17 alpha-estradiol
  - −17 beta-dihydroequilin

Other interesting facts:

- Premarin contains horse estrogens, equilin and equilenin, and additives that are synthetic. These additives and coatings may cause their own side effects including: burning in the urinary tract, allergies, joint aches, and pains.[422]

- Synthetic estrogens contain many forms of estrogen that do not fit into the estrogen receptors in your body.[551] What happens to the estrogens that do not fit into your receptors? No one knows!

- Your own estradiol molecules are eliminated from your body within a few hours. Conversely, equilin (estrogen derived from the urine of horses) has been shown to stay in your body for up to 13 weeks.[420] This is due to the fact that your enzymes are designed to metabolize your own estrogen and not equilin.[421]

How you take estrogen is also important. I recommend giving estrogen only by the *transdermal* route. This is through your skin.

Estrogen given by mouth can:[472, 550]

- Increase blood pressure
- Increase triglycerides
- Increase estrone (E1, see the chapter on natural estrogen.)
- Cause gallstones
- Can elevate liver enzymes
- Can decrease growth hormone (The hormone that keeps you youthful.)
- Interrupts tryptophan metabolism and consequently serotonin metabolism[268] (Serotonin keeps you calm and happy.)
- Increases sex hormone binding globulin (Can decrease testosterone.)
- Increases carbohydrate cravings[98]
- Increases weight gain[98]

Consequently, estrogen creams are the preferred method of replacing this hormone that has so many functions in your body.

The following chapters will look at what kind of estrogens your system makes, natural estrogens, how estrogens are metabolized, and eliminated from your body.

Summary

- Estrogen has 400 crucial functions in your body. *You need estrogen for optimal health.*

- The amount of estrogen you have is important. Too little or too much can cause symptoms or disease.

- *Synthetic estrogen is not the same chemical structure of estrogen that your own body makes. Therefore, synthetic estrogen does not fit into your estrogen receptors in your body.*

- Synthetic estrogens take a long time to be eliminated from your system.

- Synthetic estrogens have coatings and additives which may cause a problem.

- The preferred method for the administration of estrogen is transdermally (through the skin).

- Diet affects estrogen production and use.

Natural Estrogens

The potency of synthetic estrogen is about 200 times that of natural *estradiol.*[534] Therefore if you are taking a synthetic estrogen it may be more than your body needs. *Natural means biologically identical to the same chemical structure that your own body makes.*

Your body makes many kinds of estrogens. *There are three main estrogens:*

- E1 called estrone
- E2 called estradiol
- E3 called estriol

Estrone (E1)

Estrone is the main estrogen your body makes post-menopausally. *High levels stimulate breast and uterine tissue and many researchers believe it may be related to an increased risk of breast and uterine cancer.*[535, 210]

Before menopause estrone is made by your ovaries, adrenal glands, liver, and fat cells. Estrone, *pre-menopausally,* is converted to estradiol in your ovaries. *Postmenopausally,* little estrone becomes estradiol since your ovaries stop working. Estrone, in later years, is then made in your fat cells and to a lesser degree in your liver and adrenal glands.[211] Therefore, the more body fat you have the more estrone you make. Consequently, obese women have an increased estrone to estradiol ratio.[470] Also, routine alcohol consumption decreases ovarian hormone levels and shifts your estrogen to estrone.[218, 469]

Estradiol (E2)

Estradiol is the strongest estrogen. *It is 12 times stronger than estrone and 80 times stronger than estriol.* It is the main estrogen your body produces before menopause. Most of estradiol is made in your ovaries. *High levels of E2 are associated with an increased risk of breast and uterine cancer.* Estradiol is the estrogen you lose at menopause. However, two-thirds of postmenopausal women up to the age of 80 continue to make some estradiol.[141] Estradiol levels are lower in women who have had a surgical procedure that affected their ovaries. In other words, even if you had a *tubal ligation* or a *partial hysterectomy* (ovaries are left in), you may still have a decrease in your hormonal function and have menopausal symptoms. (See the chapter on surgical menopause.)[209]

Functions of estradiol in your body:[215]

- Helps maintain potassium levels
- Helps absorption of calcium, magnesium, zinc
- Increases HDL (good cholesterol)
- Decreases LDL (bad cholesterol)
- Decreases total cholesterol
- Decreases triglycerides (transdermal administration only)
- Decreases platelet stickiness (why people take an aspirin every day)
- Increases growth hormone[216]
- Increases serotonin
- Helps maintain your bones
- Increases endorphins
- Improves sleep
- Decreases fatigue
- Works as an antioxidant[217]
- Helps maintain memory

Estriol (E3)

Estriol has a much less stimulating effect on the breast and uterine lining than estrone or estradiol. *Estriol has been shown not to promote breast cancer and considerable evidence exists to show that it protects against it.* In Europe estriol has been used for many years.[355, 356, 2, 293]

Functions of estriol in your body:

- Estriol has been found to be effective at controlling symptoms of menopause, including hot flashes, insomnia, and vaginal dryness.[344, 394, 395]

- Estriol helps your gut maintain a favorable environment for the growth of good bacteria (lactobacilli) and helps reduce pathogenic bacteria.[6]

- Estriol benefits the vaginal lining.[536]

- Estriol increases HDL (the good cholesterol) and decreases LDL (the bad cholesterol).[357]

- Estriol may help restore the proper pH of the vagina and consequently help prevent urinary tract infections.[537]

- It has been used to treat breast cancer.[5]

- Estriol blocks estrone by occupying the estrogen receptor sites on your breast cells.

Asian and vegetarian women have high levels of estriol and much lower rates of breast cancer.[4]

Estriol, (E3) does not however have the bone, heart, or brain protection of estradiol (E2).[212, 471] Therefore, I usually prescribe 20% estradiol and 80% estriol to my patients. This is called bi-est and is a prescription that a compounding pharmacist can formulate for you. Any percentage can be used of these two estrogens since the dosage is individualized.

It is also necessary that you have your levels of all three estrogens measured before you begin HRT, and regularly thereafter, to help you doctor maintain you on the right amount of each type of estrogen.

Summary

- Your body makes three main estrogens:
  - E1 called estrone. Many researchers believe it may be related to an increase in breast and uterine cancer.
  - E2 called estradiol. It helps maintain your memory, bone health, and aids in protecting you from heart disease.
  - *E3 called estriol. Considerable evidence exists to show that it may protect against breast cancer.*
- Have your physician measure all three types of estrogens.
- It is important for optimal health that your HRT be comprised of estradiol and estriol (bi-est) and *not* contain estrone.
- Estradiol *alone* may be too strong of an estrogen to use as hormone replacement, plus the protective affects of estriol are not present.

Estrogen Metabolism

There is a growing body of research showing that it is not simply the amount of total estrogen circulating in your body that is critical to your health. How estrogen is broken down, or metabolized, in the body may also play an important role in the cause of a variety of estrogen-dependent conditions including: osteoporosis, autoimmune disorders, and cancer.

After menopause, the metabolism of estrogen can change. Consequently you may respond differently to estrogen.[175]

Estrogen is metabolized in your body in the following ways:

Two major competing pathways
- 2-hydroxyestrone
- 16-hydroxyestrone

One minor pathway
- 4-hydroxyestrone

2-hydroxyestrone is sometimes called the "good" estrogen.[446] It does *not* stimulate your cells to divide which can cause damage to your DNA and cause tumor growth.[447] Furthermore, by latching onto available estrogen cell receptors, 2-hydroxyestrone may exhibit a blocking action that prevents stronger estrogen products from gaining a foothold into your cells. Therefore, 2-hydroxyestrone is suggested to be anti-cancerous.[382]

The other major pathway whereby estrogen is metabolized is16-hydroxyestrone. This metabolite is much more active and powerful. It has a strong stimulatory effect. 16-hydroxyestrone binds strongly to special receptors inside your cells that can increase the rate of DNA synthesis and cell multiplication.[448] *Consequently, 16-hydroxyestrone is proposed to have significant estrogenic activity and to be associated with an increased risk of breast cancer.*[379, 369, 370, 371, 372, 373, 240, 345, 380, 381, 84] Furthermore, 16-hydroxyestrone permanently binds to the estrogen receptor. Other estrogens attach briefly and then are released.[300] This may also be a reason why 16-hydroxyestrone is associated with a higher rate of cancer.

Therefore, if you metabolize a larger proportion of endogenous (inside your body) and exogenous (outside your body) estrogen through the 16-hydroxy pathway you may be at higher risk for breast cancer than if you breakdown more estrogen through the 2-hydroxy pathway.[618]

Recent studies have shown that *low* 2/16 hydroxy estrogen ratios are associated with breast cancer. One study of postmenopausal women who went on to develop breast cancer had a 15% lower 2/16 hydroxy estrogen ratio than those in control groups.[244] Likewise, in women who already have breast cancer, the survival rate is greater in women with higher ratios.[139, 337]

A minor pathway of estrogen metabolism is 4-hydroxyestrone. *It may also enhance cancer development.* 4-hydroxyestrone may directly damage DNA by causing breaks in the molecular strands of DNA.[301] The 4-hydroxy estrogens, furthermore, have the ability to convert to metabolites that react with DNA and cause mutations that can be carcinogenic (cause cancer).[620] Also, 4-hydroxyestrone is present in greater quantities if you are deficient in methionine and folic acid.

Equine estrogens, such as Premarin, increase metabolism into 4-hydroxyestrones.[444, 619] Studies have shown that 4-hydroxyestrone from equine (horse) estrogen, causes mutagenic damage five times more rapidly than the normal 4-hydroxy estrogens.[621]

Therefore, the metabolism of estrogen via the 2-hydroxy pathway is of critical importance in lowering your risk of cellular damage (cancer).

It is consequently very important to know the levels of 2-hydroxy and 16-hydroxyestrone as well as the ratio between these two metabolites. The goal is to normalize your estrogen metabolism. Therefore, have your doctor measure your urinary metabolites of 2-hydroxy and 16-hydroxyestrone. Follow-up testing is also suggested to assess the clinical impact of dietary and lifestyle changes as well as HRT. Even if you are not on HRT you should have your 2/16 hydroxyestrone levels measured to see if you are at risk. Then modify your diet accordingly.[243] (See the appendix under Great Smokies Diagnostic Laboratory which provides this kind of testing.)

What can raise your good (2-hydroxyestrone) estrogen levels?

- Moderate exercise[374, 308]
- Cruciferous vegetables (See the end of this chapter.)[135, 136, 137, 138, 340, 36, 386, 339, 130, 131, 132, 459]
- Flax[442, 377, 457, 458, 398]
- Soy[376, 461]
- Kudzu
- Indole-3-carbinol taken as a supplement[367, 388, 342] (It has been shown to induce the enzyme P450A1 which is responsible for the formation of 2-hydroxyestrone.) Daily dose is 200 to 300 mg.
- High protein diet[375, 384]
- Omega-3-fatty acids[389, 460, 443]
- B6, B12, and folate are important in supporting the 2-hydroxyestrone pathway[129, 239]

All of these have shown to increase the 2/16 ratio significantly, thus, reducing the risk of estrogen dependent health problems by shifting estrogen metabolism toward the less active 2-hydroxyestrone pathway.

There are two other factors that affect how your body metabolizes estrogen. The first is obesity.

Obesity increases the action of estrogens in three ways:[363]

- Estrogen production and storage occurs in your fat cells.[364, 366]
- Concentrations of sex hormone binding globulin are decreased if you are heavy. This increases the amount of unbound estrogen available for usage by your body.[365]
- Obesity decreases 2-hydroxyestrone and increases 16-hydroxyestrone production.[362, 367]

The second factor is the presence of xenoestrogens. Researchers have identified fifty chemicals that imitate estrogen.[359] These are called xenoestrogens. They are toxic to your body.[85, 86, 271] (See also the chapter on detoxification.)

Sources of xenoestrogens:

- Pesticides
- Synthetic hormones fed to animals
- Plastics
- Cosmetics

In summary, these xenoestrogens influence the ratio of 2/16 hydroxy and may account for an increase in breast cancer.[245, 246]

Indole-3-Carbinol

In order for estrogen to be produced through the 2-hydroxy estrone pathway (the "good estrogen"), your body uses indole-3-carbinol.[623] It is present in cruciferous vegetables.

Vegetables that contain indole-3-carbinol are:

- Broccoli
- Brussels sprouts
- Cabbage
- Cauliflower
- Collard
- Bok choy
- Horseradish
- Kale
- Mustard seed
- Radishes
- Rutabaga
- Turnip
- Watercress

Interesting facts about indole-3-carbinol:

- Studies have shown that people given indole-3-carbinol demonstrated a 50 to 75% elevation in the good metabolism of estrogen.[53]

- If you overcook your vegetables, it destroys the indole-3-carbinol.[303] Therefore, it is best to eat them raw or lightly steamed.
- Antacids interfere with the absorption of indole-3-carbinol.[302, 396] Consequently, I do not recommend the long-term use of any antacid. I do suggest a group of herbs instead: Corydalis yanhusuo tuber, Astragalus root, Tienchi ginseng root, Zhejiang fritillary bulb, Chinese licorice root, Gambir leaf and stem, Brown's lily bulb, Bletilla root, and Sepia (cuttlefish shell). Rather than neutralizing the stomach acid production, they nourish and protect the mucosal layer of the stomach. (They are manufactured together under the name of Ulcinex by Metagenics, see the appendix for availability).
- Indole-3-carbinol may help protect obese women from the effect of excessive estrogen production.[622]

Summary

How you metabolize estrogen is important.

- The 2-hydroxy estrogens are believed to be the 'good estrogens' and are suggested to be anti-cancerous.
- The 16 and 4-hydroxy estrogens are believed to be associated with an increased risk of breast cancer.
- Equine estrogens such as Premarin increase 4-hydroxy estrogens.
- Diet, nutrients, and moderate exercise can increase your good estrogens.
- Foods high in indole-3-carbinol or supplementation of this nutrient is one of the best ways to increase good (2-hydroxy) estrogen production.
- Long-term use of antacids can interfere with the absorption of indole-3-carbinol.
- Have your doctor measure your 2-hydroxy and 16-hydroxy-estrone levels.

Estrogen and Your Brain

Estrogen has many protective affects on your brain.[270] Without estrogen, your memory usually declines.

Estrogen has the following affects on your brain:[8, 9, 10, 174, 95, 126, 127, 601, 409, 410, 411, 412, 392, 393, 313, 314, 349, 350, 270]

- Increases blood flow
- Increases glucose and oxygen to your neurons
- Regulates membrane channels
- Keeps the blood-brain barrier working
- Protects neurons
- Decreases the seizure threshold
- Increases excitability
- Affects gene expression
- Increases serotonin effect
- Increases norepinephrine effect
- Increases dopamine
- Decreases dopamine receptor sensitivity
- Increases the production of choline acetyltransferase needed for the production of acetylcholine your main neurotransmitter (Neurotransmitters help your brain cells communicate.)
- Increases GABA (calming neurotransmitter)
- Affects brain development and aging
- Increases sensitivity to nerve growth factor which stimulates the growth of dendrites and axons in your brain

- Improves the function of your neurons
- Decreases neuronal generation of Alzheimer's beta amyloid peptides (decreases the risk of developing Alzheimer's disease)

Results of several studies reveal that estrogen helps maintain your memory:

- Estrogen use in postmenopausal women may delay the beginning and decrease the risk of developing Alzheimer's disease.[76, 77]
- Women on estrogen are less than half as likely to get Alzheimer's disease than women who do not take estrogen.[11, 12]
- Estrogen use helps maintain cognitive function and maintain your ability to learn new things.[13, 41]
- A Stanford University study showed that name recall was better in women who took estrogen.[49]
- McGill University in Canada also found that women taking estrogen had better verbal memory than women not taking HRT.[50]
- A recent study conducted on 1,889 older women in Utah revealed that women who had taken HRT were 40% less likely to develop Alzheimer's disease. Furthermore, the longer they were on hormone replacement therapy the lower was their risk.[636]

In short, estrogen helps maintain your memory.[94, 146, 147, 148] For a more in depth look at this important subject, read *Menopause and the Mind,* by Claire Warga.

Estrogen not only helps maintain memory, it is also a neuroactive hormone that reacts with receptors in your brain to modulate serotonin activity. A rapid change in estrogen levels can lead to decreased serotonin levels. This can cause depression.

In summary, estrogen has many protective affects on your brain including maintaining your memory, decreasing the incidence of Alzheimer's disease, and lowering the rate of depression.

Estrogen Receptor Modulators

Selective estrogen receptor modulators, called SERMs, are a type of hormone replacement therapy. There are endogenous estrogen receptor modulators such as estriol (E3) which are made inside your body. There are also exogenous estrogen receptor modulators which are from external sources like phytoestrogens (plant sources) and pharmaceutical medications like Tamoxifen.

Tamoxifen (Nolvadex) is used for women who have had cancer to help prevent a recurrence. It works by blocking estrogen's effects on your breast tissue since it occupies cellular receptor sites for estrogen. Tamoxifen, however, does not block estrogen's affects elsewhere in your body. Consequently, it can double or triple your risk of cancer of the uterus. It also increases your risk of blood clots.[553]

Raloxifene (Evista) is also a SERM. It has selective estrogen activity for bones. It has been shown to decrease your risk for breast cancer. It can increase bone density up to 20% but that is *less* than the protection provided by hormone replacement therapy. A side effect of raloxifene is hot flashes.[554]

The SERMs decrease total cholesterol by 5% and LDL (bad cholesterol) by 10%. However, they are not very effective in lowering triglycerides and do not increase HDL (good cholesterol) as well as standard hormone replacement therapy.[555] *Furthermore, the two designer estrogens, raloxifene (Evista) and tamoxifen (Nolvadex) are not neuroprotective for the brain. 315 Consequently, they will not have the same positive effect on your memory and mood as prescription natural estrogen replacement does.*

Progesterone

Progesterone is one of your sex hormones and is made in your ovaries before menopause. After menopause, some progesterone is made in your adrenal glands.

The following are symptoms of decreased progesterone:
- Anxiety
- Depression
- Irritability
- Mood swings
- Insomnia
- Pain and inflammation
- Osteoporosis
- Decreased HDL
- Excessive menstruation

Causes of low progesterone levels are:
- Impaired production
- Low luteinizing hormone (LH)
- Increased prolactin production
- Stress[65]
- Antidepressants[67]
- Excessive arginine consumption[68]
- Sugar[69]
- Saturated fat[70]
- Deficiency of vitamins A, B6, C, zinc[71, 72]
- Decreased thyroid hormone

Synthetic progesterone is called progestin. It is very different from natural progesterone since it does *not* have the same chemical structure as the progesterone that your body makes on its own. Natural progesterone is biologically identical to what you produce. *Consequently, progestins do not reproduce the actions of natural progesterone.*[352]

Let's first look at progestins (synthetic progesterone). Progestins are contained in birth control pills, Provera, and Prempro, for example.

***The following are* side effects *of progestins (synthetic progesterone) that do* not *occur with natural progesterone:*[475, 107, 164]**

- Increases appetite[183]
- Weight gain[223]
- Fluid retention
- Irritability
- Depression
- Headache
- Decreases energy
- Bloating
- Breast tenderness
- Decreases sexual interest
- Rash
- Acne
- Hair loss
- Nausea
- Insomnia
- Breakthrough bleeding/spotting
- Interferes with your body's own production of progesterone
- Does not help balance estrogen
- Remains in your body longer
- Can cause spasm of your coronary (heart) arteries[563]
- Stops the protective affects estrogen has on your heart[43, 564, 533, 353, 354]
- Attaches to many of your body's receptor sites, not just your progesterone receptors (Long-term affects of this are unknown.)[44]

- Cannot help make estrogen and testosterone
- May make the symptoms of progesterone loss worse
- Increases LDL (bad cholesterol)
- Decreases HDL (good cholesterol)
- Protects only the uterus from cancer[108, 109]
- Counteracts many of the positive effects of estrogen on serotonin[269]

A recent study has shown that the use of synthetic progesterone increases the risk of breast cancer by 800% as compared to the use of estrogen alone.[433, 180, 181, 111] Furthermore, an article published in the *Journal of the American Medical Association* discussed a risk of breast cancer that was predicted to rise by nearly 80% after 10 years of use of estrogen-progestin (synthetic) HRT and 160% after 20 years.[112]

Likewise, Dr. Stephen Sinatra, a well-known cardiologist, states in his book, *Heart Sense for Women*, "I have found that synthetic progestins can lead to serious cardiac side effects in my patients, including shortness of breath, fatigue, chest pain, and high blood pressure."[562]

Progesterone (natural) affects not seen with progestins:[617]

- Helps balance estrogen
- Leaves your body quickly
- Helps you sleep
- Natural calming effect[19]
- Lowers high blood pressure
- Helps your body use and eliminate fats
- Lowers cholesterol
- May protect against breast cancer
- Increases scalp hair
- Normalizes libido
- Helps balance fluids in the cells
- Increases the beneficial effects of estrogens on blood vessel dilation in atherosclerotic plaques (hardening of the arteries)[17, 390, 391]

- Has an anti-proliferative effect (decreases the rate of cancer) on all progesterone receptors, not just the ones in the uterus.[108, 109]
- Does not change the good affect estrogen has on blood flow[564]
- Increases metabolic rate[494]
- Natural diuretic
- Natural antidepressant

Affects both *progestins (synthetic progesterone) and natural progesterone have in common:*
- Builds bone[413]
- Helps thyroid hormone function
- Protects against fibrocystic breast disease
- Protects against endometrial cancer
- Normalizes zinc and copper levels

Affects of too much *progesterone, (synthetic or natural).*[221, 18, 115, 505, 506]

- Increases fat storage
- Decreases glucose tolerance (May predispose you to diabetes.)
- Increases cortisol
- Increases insulin resistance
- Increases appetite
- Increases carbohydrate cravings
- Relaxes the smooth muscles of the gut[222] (This can cause bloating, fullness, and constipation. It can also contribute to gallstones).
- Suppresses immune system[231]
- Causes incontinence (leaky bladder)[539]
- Causes your ligaments to relax and can cause backaches, leg aches, and achy hips[230]
- Decreases growth hormone[234]
- Increases insulin
- Increases cortisol (See chapter on cortisol.)[234]

It is clear from this discussion, that natural progesterone offers a safer approach to HRT than synthetic progesterone (progestin).[110] It is also very important that you have your levels of progesterone measured before you begin HRT and then on a regular basis to confirm that you are on an optimal dose for you. (See the chapter on saliva testing.)

Do you need progesterone if you have had a complete hysterectomy? The answer is simply, yes, since natural progesterone has the many positive affects on your body just discussed.

Progesterone can be prescribed as a pill or a topical cream. A compounding pharmacist would then fill your prescription. It is made from an extract of soy beans or yams. Your compounded formulation of progesterone will have an enzyme added to convert the diosgenin in the yam into progesterone. Over-the-counter progesterone frequently does not contain this enzyme.[161]

If one of your main symptoms is insomnia, then choose the pill form which affects the GABA receptors in your brain.[19] GABA is an amino acid that acts as a neurotransmitter. It has a calming effect on your brain and allows you to sleep.[233] Natural progesterone is available also as Prometrium. This is made from peanut oil. The absorption rate of oral progesterone increases as you age, consequently, you need less medication as you grow older.[538]

Lastly, adrenaline also interacts with progesterone. *Adrenaline surges, which occur with stress, can block progesterone receptors.* This can prevent progesterone from being used effectively in your body.[415]

Summary

- Natural progesterone is a hormone that helps with your mood. Anxiety, irritability, insomnia, mood swings, and depression, as well as many other symptoms, are helped by progesterone.
- Synthetic progesterone, called progestin, has many side effects and does not function the same way in your body as natural progesterone.
- *Progestins (synthetic) stop the protective effects of estrogen on your heart. Natural progesterone is synergistic and increases the protective affects of estrogen on your heart.*
- If you have had a hysterectomy you may still need progesterone.
- It is important that you have your levels of progesterone measured before you begin HRT and then on a regular basis to confirm that you are on an optimal dose for you.
- *Stress increases adrenaline which can block progesterone receptors and prevent progesterone from being used effectively in your body.*
- If you take *only* progesterone and *not* estrogen (and your body is deficient in estrogen) this may predispose you to diabetes.
- If you have insomnia, then choose the pill form of progesterone which will help you sleep better than progesterone applied to you skin.

Estrogen/ Progesterone Ratio

As you have already seen, there is an increased risk of breast cancer if estrogen metabolism favors the 16-hydroxyestrone pathway. There is also a higher risk for breast cancer if you have a low progesterone to estrogen ratio.[507] This means that estrogen is unopposed, i.e., out of balance with progesterone.

Important facts about the estrogen/progesterone ratio:

- Progesterone and estradiol (estrogen) work together in your body. Estradiol lowers body fat by decreasing lipoprotein lipase, an enzyme, in your fat cells. Progesterone increases body fat storage by increasing lipoprotein lipase.[224]

- Estrogen and progesterone work together to control your body's release of insulin. Progesterone decreases insulin sensitivity and causes insulin resistance. *Women with diabetes need to use the least amount of progesterone as possible.*[255] Estradiol (E2) increases insulin sensitivity and improves glucose tolerance.

- A progesterone to estrogen ratio that is too high in progesterone will breakdown protein and muscle tissue.[228] *This will make diseases like fibromyalgia worse.*

Prolonged use of progesterone without *adequate estrogen will do the following:*[227]

- Increase weight gain
- Increase total cholesterol
- Decrease HDL (good cholesterol)
- Increase LDL (bad cholesterol)
- Increase triglycerides
- Increase insulin resistance/ predispose you to diabetes
- Cause depression
- Cause fatigue
- Decrease libido

Testosterone

Androgens are commonly called "male" hormones. They are testosterone, DHEA (dehydroepiandrosterone), and androstenedione.

This chapter will focus on testosterone. Testosterone is made in your adrenal glands and ovaries. As you age your ovaries produce less testosterone. One percent of the testosterone that you make is free, the rest is bound to sex hormone binding globulin. Women with increased androgens have more free testosterone. Therefore it is important to measure salivary hormone levels (amount of free) and not only blood levels which measure both free and bound testosterone.

Testosterone does the following things in your body:
- Increases sexual interest (86% of women state they have a decrease in sexual interest with menopause.)[21]
- Increases sense of emotional well-being, self-confidence, and motivation[497]
- Increases muscle mass and strength
- Helps maintain memory[249]
- Stimulates the growth of pubic hair and underarm hair at puberty
- Increases muscle tone so your skin does not sag[498]
- Decreases excess body fat
- Decreases bone deterioration and helps maintain bone strength[499]
- Elevates norepinephrine in the brain which has the same effect as taking a tricyclic antidepressant[250]

The following are symptoms of testosterone loss:

- Muscle wasting despite adequate calorie and protein intake
- Weight gain and decline in muscle tone
- Fatigue, decreased energy
- Low self-esteem
- Decreased HDL (good cholesterol)[500]
- Decreased sex drive
- Mild depression
- Less dreaming
- Dry, thin skin, with poor elasticity
- Loss of pubic hair
- Thinning and dry hair
- Droopy eyelids
- Sagging cheeks
- Thin lips
- Hypersensitive, hyper-emotional states
- Anxiety

Low testosterone is due to the following:

- Menopause
- Childbirth
- Chemotherapy
- Surgical menopause[24]
- Adrenal stress or burnout
- Endometriosis
- Depression
- Psychological trauma
- Birth control pills
- Cholesterol lowering medications called HMG-CoA-reductase inhibitors, such as Lipitor, Mevacor, Zocor, Pravachol, and others are all anti-androgens (will lower testosterone)[510]

What can you do to increase testosterone?
● Decrease calorie intake
● Increase protein in your diet
● Take the amino acids arginine, leucine, glutamine
● Exercise
● Get enough sleep
● Lose weight
● Practice stress reduction
● Take zinc if you are deficient (Zinc is needed for the metabolism of testosterone.)

New research is showing that in order for testosterone to work well, estradiol must also be optimized. Without enough estrogen, testosterone cannot attach to your brain receptors. *Therefore, estrogen plays a role in how well testosterone works in your body.*[251]

If testosterone is given with estradiol it lowers your cardiac risk.[540, 541] *If given alone, testosterone and DHEA increase plaque formation in your heart vessels which increases your risk for a heart attack.* If testosterone and DHEA are given with estrogen, they have a beneficial effect on your arterial walls.[248]

Prescription natural testosterone is the preferred method of testosterone replacement. Methyltestosterone (synthetic) has been suggested to be carcinogenic to your liver (can cause cancer).[190, 20, 477] Natural testosterone is effective as a pill or a cream. If used as a cream, you need to rotate application sites. If you put it on the same location all of the time (for example your right thigh), you will have an increase in hair growth there. Unfortunately, this does not work to re-grow the hair on your head.

You can have too much testosterone. Excess androgen production is usually due to over-production by your adrenal glands not your ovaries. Androgen dominance is the most common hormonal disorder found in women.[168] Almost 10% of all women have had some kind of androgen imbalance.

The following are symptoms of increased testosterone:[169]

- Anxiety
- Depression
- Changes in memory
- Fatigue
- Hypoglycemia
- Salt and sugar cravings
- Agitation
- Anger
- Facial hair
- Acne/oily skin
- Increase in insulin resistance
- Decrease in HDL (good cholesterol)
- Irregular periods
- Infertility
- Weight gain (apple body shape)
- Fluid retention
- Mood swings
- Hair loss
- Unwanted hair growth
- Increased risk of breast cancer[171]

What can you do to lower testosterone?

- Saw palmetto
- Glucophage

Reduction of testosterone hormone should be done only with the guidance of a physician.

As you can see, replacement of testosterone, and regulation of the appropriate amount of testosterone in your body are required for you to have optimum health.

Summary

- Women need testosterone if they are deficient.
- Estrogen is needed to help testosterone work.
- Testosterone should be given *with* estrogen. *If given alone, testosterone can increase your risk of heart disease.*
- Natural testosterone is a better preparation. Synthetic testosterone has been linked to cancer of the liver.
- Excessive testosterone can cause symptoms and disease.
- Salivary testing is the preferred method of measuring your levels of testosterone.

DHEA

DHEA is a hormone made by your adrenal glands. A small amount is also made in your brain and skin. DHEA production declines with age starting in your late twenties. By the age of 70 you only make one-fourth of the amount you made earlier. DHEA makes your other sex hormones, estrogen, progesterone, and testosterone.

The function of DHEA in your body:[417]
● Decreases cholesterol
● Decreases formation of fatty deposits
● Prevents blood clots
● Increases bone growth
● Promotes weight loss
● Increases brain function
● Increases sense of well being
● Helps you deal with stress
● Supports your immune system
● Helps your body repair itself and maintain tissues
● Decreases allergic reactions

Low DHEA can be due to:[25]
● Menopause
● Decreased production
● Stress
● Aging
● Smoking (Nicotine inhibits the production of an enzyme, 11-beta-hydroxylase, which is needed to make DHEA.)[150, 151]

Replacement of DHEA can:[283]

- Increase muscle strength and lean body mass
- Activate immune function
- Increase quality of life
- Improve sleep
- Increase feeling of wellness
- Decrease joint soreness
- Increase sensitivity of insulin
- Decrease triglycerides
- Stop the damaging effects of stress

DHEA has been shown to have a protective effect against cancer, diabetes, obesity, increased cholesterol, heart disease, and autoimmune diseases.[435, 436, 437]

You can over dose on DHEA. Women are more sensitive to the affects of DHEA and need less DHEA than men.

The following are symptoms of too much DHEA:

- Fatigue
- Anger
- Depression
- Deepening of voice
- Insomnia
- Mood changes
- Weight gain
- Facial hair
- Acne
- Sugar cravings
- Restless sleep
- Irritability

Summary

- DHEA is another sex hormone. It makes your other sex hormones.
- Optimal replacement of DHEA helps your maintain optimal health.
- Your levels of DHEA should be measured before and after replacement.
- DHEA is a hormone and should not be taken if you are not deficient. You can over dose on DHEA.
- Women are more sensitive to the affects of DHEA and need less DHEA than men.

Cortisol

Cortisol is the only hormone in your body that increases with age. It is also one of your sex hormones. Cortisol and DHEA are both made by your adrenal glands which also make your sex hormones after menopause.

Cortisol is involved in the following ways in your body:[81, 82]

- Balancing blood sugar
- Weight control
- Immune system response
- Bone turnover rate
- Stress reaction
- Sleep
- Protein synthesis
- Mood and thoughts
- Influences testosterone/ estrogen ratio
- Influences DHEA/insulin ratio
- Affects pituitary/thyroid/ adrenal system

Stress increases cortisol as does depression and high progestin intake (birth control pills and synthetic progesterone).[255]

The following are long term consequences of elevated cortisol:[83, 260]

- Decreased immune system
- Increased osteoporosis risk
- Fatigue
- Irritability
- Sugar cravings
- Shakiness between meals
- Confusion
- Sleep disturbances
- Low energy
- Night sweats
- Binge eating
- Increased blood pressure
- Increased cholesterol
- Increased triglycerides
- Increased blood sugar
- Increased insulin/insulin resistance

- Increased infections
- Thin skin
- Easy bruising
- Muscle weakness
- Weight gain

Abnormal cortisol levels are associated with the following conditions:[80]

- Menopause
- Chronic fatigue syndrome
- Fibromyalgia
- Depression
- Impotence
- Anorexia nervosa
- Panic disorders
- PMS
- Infertility
- Sleep disorders
- Osteoporosis
- Heart disease

All of the hormones in your body work together. In order for you to have good health they all have to be balanced and at an optimal level. *If your cortisol is increased, it decreases the making of progesterone and its activity.*[143] Cortisol competes with progesterone for common receptors. Furthermore, *when cortisol is high it makes your thyroid hormone become more bound and therefore less active.*[256]

When your adrenal glands are in a state of "emergency" you do not feel well. You may reach for coffee, soft drinks, or sugar for a source of energy. This makes the situation worse. If your adrenal glands stay stimulated you cause them to weaken or *"burn out."* Then your cortisol and DHEA levels drop.

The following symptoms can then occur:

- Fatigue
- Low blood pressure
- Sensitivity to light
- Insomnia
- Digestive problems
- Emotional imbalances
- Hypoglycemia (low blood sugar)
- Decreased sexual interest

Many women enter menopause with progesterone loss due to exhaustion of their adrenal glands. Your doctor can treat you with pregnenolone (see the chapter on pregnenolone), DHEA, or cortef (cortisone) to help with adrenal burn out. Have your levels measured before you start on any of these hormones. I also use the herbs,

Cordyceps (Cordyceps sinensis), Asian ginseng (Panax ginseng) and Rhodiola (Rhodiola rosea), in my practice as adaptogens for patients with adrenal burnout. Adaptogens are biological substances found in certain plants and herbs that help the body "adapt" to stressors of various kinds. All of these herbs are combined together under the product name Adreset made by Metagenics. (For information concerning availability of this product see the appendix.)

Decreased estradiol (estrogen) is, in itself, a stressor to your body. It causes an increase in cortisol because decreased estradiol causes a decrease in optimal function of norepinephrine, serotonin, dopamine, and acetylcholine.[261] These are neurotransmitters responsible for communication between your cells.

Neurotransmitters regulate the following:
- Weight
- Appetite
- Muscle growth and repair
- Sleep
- Mood
- Memory
- Thirst
- Sexual interest
- Pain

Summary

- Cortisol is the only hormone in your body that increases with age.

- High levels of cortisol are associated with numerous symptoms and diseases including a suppressed immune system and weight gain.

- Your adrenal glands can become 'burnt out' due to over stimulation.

- *Many women enter menopause with progesterone loss due to exhaustion of their adrenal glands.*

- Herbs, pregnenolone, DHEA, and cortef are effective treatments for adrenal dysfunction.

Insulin and Your Sex Hormones

Estrogen, progesterone, DHEA, and thyroid hormones are all very important for the regulation of glucose in your body.

If insulin (your hormone that regulates glucose) becomes unresponsive or resistant, your blood sugar will rise and you can develop Type II diabetes.

Things that increase insulin:[466]

- High carbohydrate diet
- Increased stress
- Decreased estrogens
- Increased testosterone
- Insomnia
- Increased DHEA
- Decreased thyroid hormone
- Excessive progesterone
- Lack of exercise

Interesting facts:

- Estradiol (E2) helps improve the body's responsiveness to insulin.[467]
- High insulin levels are associated with higher testosterone and lower estrogen levels in women.[57]
- Elevated insulin levels can decrease the synthesis of DHEA, your hormone that makes your other sex hormones.[58] This is due to insulin's affect on an adrenal enzyme, 17, 20-lyase, that makes DHEA.[59]
- Insulin increases your ratio of fat to muscle. Consequently, an increase in insulin decreases fat burning.[466]
- A recent study revealed that women who have heart disease, HRT reduced the incidence of diabetes by 35%.[637]

Thyroid Hormone

It is common for thyroid problems to begin to appear at menopause. Your ovaries have thyroid receptors. Your thyroid gland has ovarian receptors. Therefore the loss of estradiol and testosterone from your ovaries that occurs at menopause can change your thyroid status.

An imbalance of your thyroid hormone can affect every metabolic function in your body. Your thyroid gland is your body regulator. It regulates energy and heat production, growth, tissue repair and development, and stimulates protein synthesis. Furthermore, thyroid hormone modulates carbohydrates, protein and fat metabolism, vitamin uses, digestion, function of the mitochondria (energy makers of your cells), muscle and nerve action, blood flow, hormone excretion, oxygen utilization, and sexual function to list just some its uses.

- TSH (thyroid stimulating hormone) is made in your pituitary gland located in your brain.

- T4 is made in your thyroid gland and is called thyroxine.

- T3 is made in other tissues and is called triiodothyronine.

Your body produces T4 and T3. T4 is 80% of the thyroid gland's production. Most of T4 is changed into T3 in your liver or kidneys. T3 is five times more active than T4. T4 can also be converted to reverse T3 which is an inactive form. Your body also makes T2. T2 increases the metabolic rate of your muscles and fat tissue.[429]

The following are symptoms of low thyroid production (hypothyroidism):

- Depression
- Weight gain
- Constipation
- Headaches
- Brittle nails
- Rough, dry skin
- Menstrual irregularities
- Fluid retention
- Poor circulation
- Elbow keratosis
- Diffuse hair loss
- Slow speech
- Anxiety/panic attacks
- Decreased memory
- Inability to concentrate
- Muscle and joint pain
- Reduced heart rate
- Slow movements
- Morning stiffness
- Puffy face
- Swollen eyelids
- Decreased sexual interest
- Cold intolerance
- Cold hands and feet
- Swollen legs, feet, hands, abdomen
- Insomnia
- Fatigue
- Low body temperature
- Hoarse, husky voice
- Low blood pressure
- Muscle weakness
- Agitation
- Sparse, coarse, dry hair
- Dull facial expression
- Yellowish color of the skin
- Muscle cramps
- Drooping eyelids
- Carpel tunnel syndrome

Other interesting facts about hypothyroidism:

- Thyroid hormones also affect muscle metabolism. If your thyroid is not functioning optimally then you do not build muscle.

- Low thyroid hormone levels directly cause low pregnenolone levels in hypothyroid patients.[440] (See chapter on pregnenolone.)

- Mild thyroid dysfunction is associated with heart disease.[103, 104]

- Decreased T3 production will cause less cholesterol to be removed from your blood which causes an elevation of LDL (bad cholesterol).[101, 426] People with low thyroid levels have raised cholesterol levels 10 to 50% higher than people with normal thyroid function.102

● Many people with fibromyalgia have hypothyroidism.[433]

When your doctor sends you for thyroid studies your entire thyroid panel should be measured. This includes your free T3, free T4, reverse T3, TSH, and thyroid antibodies.

If your antibodies are too high they can stop thyroid hormone from attaching to your thyroid receptors. Consequently you can get symptoms of decreased thyroid function even when your blood levels are adequate. Thyroid antibodies can be elevated due to trauma, poor function of your gut, inflammation, and thyroid degeneration.

Many factors affect how your body produces T3 and T4.

Some factors that cause decreased production of T4 include a deficiency in:

● Zinc
● Copper
● Vitamins A, B2, B3, B6, C

Furthermore, your body needs to be able to convert T4 to T3, the more active form. The conversion of T4 to T3 requires an enzyme called 5'diodinase.

Elements that affect 5'diodinase production:[34, 35, 36, 37]

● Selenium deficiency
● Stress
● Cadmium, mercury, or lead toxicity
● Starvation
● Inadequate protein intake
● High carbohydrate diet
● Elevated cortisol
● Chronic illness
● Decreased kidney or liver function

Other factors also cause an inability to convert T4 to T3:[427, 186, 106]

Nutrient deficiencies:

- Iodine
- Iron
- Selenium
- Zinc
- Vitamins A, B2, B6, B12

Medications:

- Beta blockers
- Birth control pills[439]
- Estrogen[439]
- Lithium
- Phenytoin
- Theophylline
- Chemotherapy

Diet:

- Cruciferous vegetables (too many)
- Low protein diet
- Low fat diet
- Low carbohydrate diet[252]
- Excessive alcohol use
- Soy[253, 254]
- Walnuts

Other:

- Aging
- Alpha-lipoic acid (too much)
- Diabetes
- Fluoride
- Lead
- Mercury[441]
- Pesticides
- Radiation
- Stress
- Surgery
- Copper excess
- Calcium excess (You can take too much calcium.)
- Dioxins
- PCB
- Inadequate production of adrenal hormones (DHEA, cortisol)
- Phtalates (chemicals added to plastics)

If you cannot convert T4 to T3 adequately you will have symptoms of thyroid hormone loss. This is also true if you have decreased T3 or increased reverse T3.

Factors associated with decreased T3 or increased reverse T3:[73]

- Increased catecholamines (epinephrine, norepinephrine)
- Increased free radicals
- Aging
- Fasting
- Stress
- Prolonged illness
- Diabetes
- Toxic metal exposure
- IL-6, TNF-alpha, IFN-2 (immune system factors)

Furthermore, things that impair your body's response to T3 will cause you to have symptoms of low thyroid. These include iron deficiency and physical inactivity.[38, 39]

There are factors that will increase the conversion of T4 to T3 if not enough T3 is being made by your body.

Factors that increase the conversion of T4 to T3:

- Selenium
- Potassium
- Iodine
- Iron
- Zinc

- High protein diet
- Ashwaganda

- Vitamins A, B2, E
- Growth hormone
- Testosterone
- Insulin
- Glucagons
- Melatonin
- Tyrosine

It is important that your doctor replace both T3 and T4 if you are diagnosed to have hypothyroidism (low thyroid levels). If you only have your T4 pathway replaced you may still experience low thyroid symptoms. Replacing T3 and T4 has been found to be more effective than replacing T4 alone.[105] One study revealed that 35% of people on T4 and T3 replacement scored better on mental agility tests. Sixty-seven percent of these people studied stated they had an improvement in mood and physical health. Likewise, benefits have been shown by adding T3 for patients already on T4. They have improved mood and brain function.[430]

Synthroid or Levothyroxine are both comprised of only T4. Armour thyroid is T3, T4, T1, T2 plus other substances that help the body convert T4 to T3 (calcitonin, selenium, and diuretic effect).[428] Some physicians feel that Armour thyroid is not consistent from dose to dose. However, there has never been a complaint to the FDA concerning the inconsistency of Armour thyroid.[431] For a lengthier discussion on thyroid disease read *Overcoming Thyroid Disorders* by Dr. David Brownstein.

Another way of replacing both thyroid pathways besides taking Armour thyroid is to add T3 (Cytomel) to T4 (Synthroid etc.).

It is also important that you check your basal body temperature if you have symptoms of hypothyroidism and you have normal blood levels of thyroid hormone. If your basal body temperature is low (below 97.4 degrees Fahrenheit) then you may benefit from a low dose of Armour thyroid even though your blood level of thyroid hormone is within normal range.

How to check your basal body temperature:

Upon awakening, place a temperature under your arm for 10 minutes and record your temperature for 5 days in a row. You cannot get out of bed before checking your temperature or your results will not be accurate.

How you respond to hormone replacement is also associated with your own unique genetic make-up. Therefore, if you are sensitive to thyroid hormone replacement you may have a genetic problem with detoxifying which will be discussed later in this book.[153, 154]

Summary

- *Hypothyroidism (low thyroid) frequently appears at menopause.*
- Your thyroid is your body regulator, therefore it needs to be functioning at an optimal level.
- *If you are taking thyroid replacement, you need T3 as well as T4.*
- Nutrition is a very important part of how well your thyroid functions.
- Medications can affect your body's ability to make thyroid hormone.
- Toxins can affect thyroid function.
- Your other hormones greatly affect how your thyroid hormone is working.
- *It is important that your doctor test your entire thyroid panel and not just your TSH to see if you are hypothyroid.*

Melatonin

Melatonin is another hormone that your body makes. It sets your body's 24-hour cycle. Melatonin is made from the amino acid tryptophan which is also used to make serotonin. Therefore, when melatonin goes up, serotonin goes down. If you eat too many high sugar carbohydrates you will make less melatonin because carbohydrates shift your amino acid balance to make more serotonin.[462]

You need B vitamins to convert melatonin from tryptophan. Therefore, if you do not have an adequate intake of vitamin B rich foods or do not take a supplement, your body may be deficient in melatonin.

Melatonin influences the following:[26, 27, 275, 594]

- Sleep
- Mood
- Stress response
- Immune function
- Release of sex hormones
- Antioxidant activity (It is more potent than vitamin C or E.)[28, 149, 273]
- Helps to prevent cancer
- Blocks estrogen from binding to estrogen receptors[278]
- Stimulates the parathyroid gland which regulates bone formation[276]
- Stimulates the production of growth hormone
- Decreases cortisol
- Increases the action of benzodiazepine medications

Other important facts about melatonin:

- *At menopause there is a decline in melatonin secretion.*[277] Therefore, you should have your melatonin levels measured.

- Recent studies are now suggesting that melatonin and testosterone regulate the synthesis of each other.[29]

- Studies have revealed that melatonin is lower in patients with heart disease than healthy people.[274]

Tryptophan (which makes melatonin) is found in fish, lamb, chicken, turkey, and pumpkin seeds. Melatonin is in rice, barley, and corn.

Other things that increase melatonin production:

- Supplementation
- Sleep
- Medication
- Exercise[31]

Factors that can decrease melatonin:[281, 594]

- Beta blockers
- Calcium channel blockers
- Alpha adrenergic blockers
- Ibuprofen
- Tranquilizers
- Aspirin
- Caffeine
- Alcohol
- Tobacco
- Electromagnetic fields[280]

Side effects of too much melatonin:

- Intense dreaming, nightmares
- Daytime sleepiness/fatigue
- Depression
- Headaches
- Increases cortisol which can increase fat storage[464]
- Suppresses serotonin which will increase your carbohydrate cravings

If you take melatonin and your levels become too high you may suppress estrogen and testosterone in your body. In contrast, if you have too little melatonin you may increase the risk of age-related diseases.[30] Consequently, it is very important to have the right amount of this hormone in your body.

Pregnenolone

Pregnenolone is a precursor to (makes) DHEA, progesterone, estrogen, testosterone, and cortisol. Your body synthesizes this hormone from cholesterol. Pregnenolone decreases with age. At age 75, most people have a 65% decline compared to age 35.[160]

Functions of pregnenolone in your body:

- Regulates the balance between excitation and inhibition in the nervous system

- Increases resistance to stress

- Improves energy both physically and mentally

- Enhances nerve transmission and memory

- Reduces pain and inflammation

- Blocks the production of acid-forming compounds

Your natural pathways of pregnenolone are blocked when you eat too much saturated fat and trans-fatty acids.[358] When this occurs you do not make the optimum amounts of your other sex hormones.

Pregnenolone is used in the treatment of arthritis, depression, memory loss, fatigue, and moodiness.

Side effects of overuse of pregnenolone are acne and drowsiness.

Prolactin

Prolactin is yet another hormone your body produces. It is made by your pituitary gland located in your brain.

Elevated prolactin can suppress your ovarian function which is responsible for the production of estradiol, progesterone, and testosterone.[207] Furthermore, prolactin can cause weight gain if elevated.[206] It can also cause breast enlargement, muscle loss, headaches, depression, and bone loss.

Things that cause an elevation of prolactin:[208]

- Menopause
- Stress
- Excessive exercise
- Hypothyroidism
- Medications:
    - SSRI anti-depressants (Prozac, Paxil, Zoloft, Celexa, Luvox)
    - Tricyclic anti-depressants
    - H2 blockers (Tagamet, Pepcid)
    - Neuroleptic medications (Haldol, Mellaril)
- Pituitary tumor

"Our bodies are exposed to an increasing number of toxic compounds in the environment as well as to a growing variety of drugs. Given these exposures, the individual's genotypic and phenotypic ability to detoxify are now recognized as key factors to overall health."

—JEFFREY BLAND, PHD

Detoxification

Estrogen synthesis, metabolism, and detoxification are of paramount importance in order to maintain optimal health.[96] Two previous chapters have discussed estrogen synthesis and metabolism. This chapter will look at detoxification.

The affect of estrogen on your body is not related solely to its function but also by how it is detoxified in the liver and other tissues. It is modified through environmental exposure, diet, and lifestyle.

Common symptoms of toxin build up include headaches, muscular aches and pains, and fatigue. Toxicity also can affect your immune, neurological, and endocrine systems.

- Immune toxicity may be a factor in asthma, allergies, skin disorders, chronic infections, and cancer.

- Neurological toxicity affects cognition, mood, and neurological function.

- Endocrine toxicity affects reproduction, menstruation, libido, metabolic rate, stress tolerance, and glucose regulation.

Important facts about your exposure to toxins:

- According to the U.S. Environmental Protection Agency, more than 4 billion pounds of chemicals were released into the ground in the year 2000, threatening our natural ground water sources.[583]

- The average American unknowingly eats about 124 pounds of additives a year.[584]

● Each year over 2.5 billion pounds of pesticides are dumped on crop lands, forests, lawns, and fields.[585]

In your environment you are exposed on a daily basis to estrogen-like compounds. These are called *xenoestrogens.* (See also the chapter on estrogens.) They are environmental compounds with estrogenic activity. Xenoestrogens can interfere with or mimic your own hormone synthesis. Consequently, they are disruptive to your own hormone production.

Your exposure to toxins is increased by:[586]
● Eating a diet high in processed foods and fat
● Drinking tap water
● Excessive consumption of caffeine containing beverages
● Excessive alcohol consumption
● Tobacco use
● Recreational drug use
● Chronic use of medication(s)
● Lack of exercise
● Liver dysfunction
● Kidney problems
● Intestinal (gut) dysfunction
● Occupational exposure
● Using pesticides, paint, and other toxic substances without adequate protective gear
● Living or working near areas of high vehicle traffic or industrial plants

How Much Toxin Load Are You Carrying?
The Detoxification Process
Detoxification is a process by which your body transforms toxins and medications into harmless molecules that can be eliminated. This process takes place primarily in the liver and to a smaller degree in other tissues.

Detoxification is largely accomplished in 2 phases:
- Phase I—Certain enzymes change toxins into intermediate compounds.
- Phase II—Other enzymes convert the intermediate compounds created in Phase I into harmless molecules that are eliminated by your body.

It is very important for you to detoxify estrogen completely in your body. This is done through phase I and phase II detoxification.

Phase I: Your First Line of Defense

In Phase I detoxification, enzymes in the cytochrome P-450 system use oxygen to modify toxic compounds, medications, and steroid hormones. This is your first line of defense for the detoxification of all environmental toxins, medications, supplements (eg., vitamins), as well as many waste products that your body produces.

Phase I occurs in the liver where estrogen goes through the cytochrome P450 system. This influences the amount of estrogen exposure to your other cells. If you do not completely detoxify the intermediates of estrogen metabolism, it can result in an *increase* in estrogen activity in your body.

Within your own genetic makeup, there are variations called single nucleotide polymorphisms, called SNPs, pronounced "snips." These SNPs in your genes code for a particular enzyme that can increase or decrease the activity of that enzyme. Both increased and decreased activity may be harmful to you. Furthermore, if you have increased Phase I clearance without increased Phase II clearance, this can lead to the build up of intermediates that may be *more toxic* than the original substance. *Decreased Phase I clearance will cause toxic accumulation in your body.* Adverse reactions to medications are often due to a decreased capacity for clearing them from your system.

Phase II Detoxification: Conjugation of Toxins and Elimination

In Phase II detoxification large water-soluble molecules are added to toxins, usually at the reactive site formed by Phase I reactions. After Phase II modifications, the body is able to eliminate the transformed toxins in the urine or the feces.

The recent completion of the Human Genome Project has made it possible to evaluate genetic variations that affect Phase I and Phase II detoxification and oxidative protection. This genetically-based test is called *Genovations* and is available through Great Smokies Diagnostic Laboratory (see appendix). Your doctor, through this kind of testing, can determine if your detoxification system in your body is working. This allows your physician to identify potential genetic trouble spots in your self-defense system *early*. Then your doctor can design precise, individualized therapy to support your detoxification. Consequently, many health problems can be *avoided* and adverse reactions to medications and supplements can be prevented *before* they happen. For example, one gene evaluated in this new profile testing, CYP3A4, affects an enzyme that your body uses to detoxify over 50% of all drugs. These medications include many antidepressants, steroid hormones (like estrogen), and cholesterol lowering medications.

This test identifies increased genetic susceptibility to:
- Adverse drug reactions
- Numerous cancers
- Neurodegenerative disorders
- Mood disorders
- Fatigue syndromes
- Fibromyalgia
- Multiple chemical sensitivity
- Oxidative stress

Adverse reactions to prescription drugs have been ranked as the fourth to the sixth leading cause of death in the United

States.[587] Each year about 100,000 Americans die from adverse reactions to medications.[588] This is more than double the number killed in motor vehicle accidents. Annual hospital costs from these reactions have been estimated to be between $1 to $4 billion.[589]

The benefits of Genovations Testing are the following:

- Reduce adverse drug reactions.
- Detect genetic susceptibility to environmental carcinogens (which are linked to 50 to 95% of cancer risk).[590]
- Uncover potential steroid hormone toxicity (occurs in up to 40% of major population segments).[591]
- Optimize drug and nutrient therapies to support healthy detoxification and overcome genetic predispositions to oxidative stress and disease.

You should consider having your detoxification pathways evaluated if you are taking hormone replacement therapy.

The detoxification process is very nutrient dependent. Phase I and Phase II enzymes are like the engines that drive the detoxification process and they are fueled by vitamins, minerals, and other key food components. Therefore, if you are undernourished, lack key vitamins or nutrients, you may not be able to deactivate estrogen properly. This can leave estrogen available to cause cell transformation in the breast and predispose you to breast cancer. *Therefore, adequate nutrition is essential for effective detoxification.*

As you have seen, genetic, biochemical, nutritional, and environmental factors can have a powerful influence over hormone replacement outcomes.

Summary

- The effect of estrogen on your body is not related solely to its synthesis and metabolism, but also how it is detoxified.

- You are exposed to toxins on a routine basis including environmental estrogens called xenoestrogens.

- *It is very important for you to detoxify estrogen completely in your body.*

- Detoxification is largely accomplished in two phases: Phase I and Phase II.

- Increased Phase I clearance without increased Phase II clearance can lead to the build up of *toxic intermediates* that may be more toxic than the original substance.

- Adequate nutrition is essential for effective detoxification.

- Consider having your detoxification pathways evaluated by *Genovations* testing through your doctor.

Osteoporosis

By the age of 60, almost one-half of the women in the U.S. will have osteoporosis.[14] One in five women will break a hip in her lifetime.[15] One-half of the women who fall and break a hip never walk again.

To maintain your bone health, your body needs calcium, magnesium, boron, manganese, and vitamins D and K.

Calcium

Numerous studies have shown that calcium supplementation can help decrease bone loss by 30 to 50%.[598] The amount needed by a peri or postmenopausal woman to prevent bone loss is 1600 mg a day. This amount includes *both* what you eat and take as a supplement.

Important facts:
- Calcium should be taken throughout the day for maximum absorption. It is best taken with meals and at bed time.
- Milk is *not* the best source of calcium since pasteurization destroys up to 32% of the available calcium.[597]
- Tums is *not* a good source of calcium intake. It is poorly absorbed.[599]
- Always use only pharmaceutical grade supplements. Lower grade products may be contaminated with lead, mercury, arsenic, aluminum, and cadmium. (For suggestions on companies that use pharmaceutical grade supplements see the appendix.)
- Vitamin C increases calcium absorption by 100%.[603]

- Calcium helps make cholesterol available to make hormones.[516]
- Calcium carbonate is not the best form of calcium to use. Calcium citrate or hydroxyappetite are now the preferred forms.[606]
- Calcium is also needed for the absorption of vitamin B12.
- You can take too much calcium.

Excess calcium supplementation can:
- Clog your arteries (predispose you to heart disease)[604]
- Block the uptake of manganese in your body
- Interfere with the absorption of magnesium
- Decrease iron absorption
- Interfere with the absorption of zinc
- Interfere with the making of vitamin K
- Cause kidney stones

The following is a list of calcium rich foods:[608, 609, 610]

- Kelp
- Brick cheese
- Barley
- Sesame seeds
- Almonds
- Shrimp
- Soybeans
- Hazelnuts
- Parsley
- Turnip greens
- Brazil nuts
- Dandelion greens
- Kale
- Sunflower seeds
- Watercress
- Garbanzo beans
- Ripe olives
- English walnuts
- Pecans
- Dates
- Dried prunes
- White beans
- Mustard greens
- Black beans
- Pinto beans
- Broccoli
- Yogurt
- Beet greens
- Tofu
- Chinese cabbage
- Eggs
- Brown rice
- Bluefish, salmon, mackerel, halibut
- Chicken
- Ground beef

Factors that decrease calcium absorption:[595, 596, 600, 601]

- High fiber cereals
- Fiber supplements (calcium should not be taken within two hours)
- Whole wheat
- Spinach
- Swiss chard
- Increased fat diet
- Increased zinc
- Diet high in breads
- Soft drinks
- White flour
- Heavy exercise
- Rhubarb
- Cocoa, chocolate

Magnesium

Magnesium is also required for bone health. Peri and post-menopausal women need 600 to 800 mg a day of magnesium. Your calcium to magnesium ratio should be about 2:1. Magnesium citrate has the best absorption rate.[607]

Role magnesium plays in your bone health:[605]

- Increases the absorption of calcium
- Activates vitamin D
- Aids in parathyroid function (decreases bone breaking down)
- Helps calcitonin function (increases the absorption of calcium)
- Activates bone-building osteoblasts
- Increases mineralization density

List of magnesium rich foods:[611, 612]

- Kelp
- Wheat bran
- Wheat germ
- Almonds
- Cashews
- Brown rice
- Corn
- Brazil nuts
- Sunflower seeds
- Sesame seeds
- Rye
- Pumpkin seeds
- Brewer's yeast
- Buckwheat
- Peanuts
- Wheat grain
- Tofu
- Coconut
- Soybeans
- Spinach, raw
- Dried figs
- Swiss chard

- Apricots, dried
- Dates
- Collard leaves
- Shrimp
- Avocados
- Cheddar cheese
- Parsley
- Prunes, dried
- Dandelion greens
- Dark green vegetables

Vitamin D

Vitamin D is needed for the absorption of calcium and the mineralization of bone. The recommended daily amount is 400 to 800 IU. Vitamin D is mainly available through sunlight. You make Vitamin D in your skin from exposure to the sun. Dairy products, fish and fish liver oils, liver, sweet potatoes, and dandelion greens also contain some vitamin D.

Vitamin K

Vitamin K helps your body maintain a hormone called osteocalcin which is needed for bone mineralization.

Sources of vitamin K:[613]
- Spinach
- Turnip greens
- Broccoli
- Green cabbage
- Tomatoes
- Liver
- Egg yolks
- Whole wheat
- Fruits
- Cheese
- Ham
- Beef

Boron

Boron is needed for calcium metabolism and it helps activate estrogen and vitamin D. Boron along with vitamin D increases the mineral content in your bone and also increases cartilage formation.[515]

Food sources of boron:[614]
- Prunes
- Raisins
- Dates
- Almonds
- Peanuts
- Hazelnuts
- Honey

Manganese

Manganese is needed for the repair of bones and connective tissue. Too much calcium can decrease the absorption of manganese.

Manganese is needed for the production of both estrogen and progesterone.[521] A decrease in manganese is also related to abnormal glucose metabolism.[522]

Sources of manganese:[615]

- Hazelnuts
- Pecans
- Avocados
- Seaweed
- Whole grains such as oatmeal, buckwheat, and whole wheat (Refined grains are a poor source of manganese.)

The following are risk factors for osteoporosis:[616, 185]

- Menopause
- Hyperthyroidism (elevated thyroid hormone)
- Parathyroid gland over production
- Vitamin D deficiency
- Calcium deficiency
- Medications
    - Dilantin and other anticonvulsants
    - Corticosteroids
    - Heparin
    - Isoniazid
    - Lasix
    - Lithium
    - Excessive thyroid medication
    - Methotrexate
- Aluminum containing antacids
- Smoking
- Alcohol
- Genetic predisposition
- Fair complexion
- Thin bone structure

- No menstrual cycle for more than 6 months
- Lack of exercise
- Caffeine
- Fluoride in drinking water[114]
- High fat diets
- Excessive zinc supplementation
- Too much vitamin A
- Soft drink use
- Long-term use of antacids

Some women inherit a gene that decreases the absorption of calcium in their bones. Therefore, your family history plays a role in your personal risk of osteoporosis. Genome testing is now available to see if you have this genetic predisposition by Great Smokies Diagnostic Laboratory under their *Genovations* testing. (See the appendix.)

Nutrients alone are not enough to prevent osteoporosis. Approximately 93% of women who do not take estrogen will have a fracture by the age of 85.[582] Estrogen maintains bone and therefore retards the progression of osteoporosis. It controls the absorption of calcium into the bone. It also stimulates the production of calcitonin which is a hormone that protects bone. Progesterone builds bone.[189] Testosterone makes the bone strong.

Deoxypridinoline (Dpd)

Researchers are now looking at bone turnover (breakdown) as a better indicator of fracture risk from osteoporosis than bone density.[334] Measuring the biochemical markers of bone turnover such as deoxypridinoline (Dpd) in the urine are a good way to accurately gauge response to hormone replacement therapy, or drug treatment, to see if it is helping your bone health. Dpd is a product of the breakdown of a kind of collagen found in your bones. When bones breakdown Dpd is eliminated in your urine. Dpd is therefore a specific marker of bone breakdown. Dpd-bone-reabsorption testing is a very effective way of measuring these levels. By doing this study your doctor can fully evaluate the status of your bones and the rate in which they are breaking down or building. (For availability of this test, see Great Smokies Diagnostic Laboratory in the appendix.) Urine levels of Dpd usually decrease within 30 days of starting estrogen therapy.[335, 336]

Summary

- To maintain your bone health, your body needs calcium, magnesium, boron, manganese, and vitamins D and K.
- Milk and Tums are not the best source of calcium intake.
- Use pharmaceutical grade supplements only.
- You can intake too much calcium.
- There are numerous causes of osteoporosis including a genetic predisposition (inherited).
- *Nutrients alone are not enough to prevent osteoporosis.* Estrogen, progesterone, testosterone, and DHEA are needed.
- Bone breakdown is a good indicator of fracture risk from osteoporosis. Dpd (biochemical markers of bone turnover) can be measured with a urine test.

Secondary Risk Factors for Heart Disease

It is important as a woman that you have your secondary risk factors of heart disease measured. These factors are homocysteine, iron (ferritin), lipoprotein(a), fibrinogen, and c-reactive protein.

Homocysteine

Homocysteine is an amino acid produced by ineffective protein metabolism that promotes free radical production.

Free radicals are molecules that lack an electron. They will go searching in your body for an electron, will find a healthy cell, and steal its electron. This kills the cell. This is one of the causes of oxidative stress that leads to heart disease. Homocysteine also elevates triglycerides and cholesterol synthesis.[284]

Studies suggest that 42% of strokes, 28% of peripheral vascular disease (causes leg pain, cramping, and loss of circulation), and approximately 30% of cardiovascular disease (heart attacks, chest pain) are directly related to elevated homocysteine levels.[565, 568, 624, 625] Furthermore, a study published in the *New England Journal of Medicine* in July 1997 showed that people with homocysteine levels below 9 were much less likely to die.[570] Another study showed that women with a history of high blood pressure and elevated homocysteine were 25 times more likely to have a heart attack or stroke.[571]

Increased homocysteine occurs with:[285]

- Menopause
- Smoking
- Hypothyroidism
- Renal failure
- Drugs
- Hereditary predisposition
- Toxins

Before menopause you have a lower homocysteine level. As you go through menopause your homocysteine levels start to rise because estrogen status is associated with homocysteine concentrations.[121] Several studies have shown that hormone replacement therapy lowers homocysteine levels as does supplementation of vitamins B6, B12, and folate.[121, 122, 123, 125, 331, 332, 333, 400, 401] *Conversely, any factor that decreases estrogen or elevates testosterone levels can increase homocysteine in both pre and postmenopausal women.*[119, 402, 403] This includes stress and the lack of exercise.[120]

High homocysteine may also be hereditary. Some people are lacking an enzyme to break down homocysteine called methylenetetrahydrofolate reductase.[567] A deficiency of this enzyme increases the need for folate in order to prevent a high homocysteine level. This occurs in 12% of the population.[287, 128] In my practice I use the active form of folic acid (L-5-MTHF) for patients who take B6, B12, and folate but still have elevated homocysteine levels. (For availability of this product, named FolaPro, see the appendix under Metagenics.)

Additionally, an elevated homocysteine level has recently been associated with the risk of memory loss.[124]

As previously stated, your body needs adequate B6, B12, and folate in order to breakdown homocysteine. B vitamins are water soluble and excessive ingestion of caffeine products, alcohol, or diuretics (water pills) will wash B vitamins out of your system. Researchers have suggested that folate supplementation could save 20,000 to 50,000 lives a year from heart disease.[572] Folate is also found in dark green leafy vegetables, beans, legumes, and oranges. Broccoli, spinach, and beets also increase the conversion of homocysteine in your body. Likewise, SAM-e (s-adenosylmethionine) will also help breakdown homocysteine. The suggested dosage is 200 to 400 mg a day.

Iron

New studies have shown that too much iron can increase your risk of heart disease. Every 1% increase in ferritin (serum iron) causes a 4% elevation in risk of heart attack.[579] Therefore, if you are no longer having menstrual cycles you do not need to take iron supplements unless instructed to do so by your doctor. Iron supplements may elevate your ferritin level and may predispose you to a heart attack. Also, your levels of iron increase after menopause, so it is a good idea to have them measured.[580]

Fibrinogen

Fibrinogen is a clot-promoting substance in your blood. If the blood levels of fibrinogen are too high it can cause a heart attack. Fibrinogen increases as estrogen decreases. Fibrinogen also elevates if you are a smoker. *Research has shown that estrogen replacement therapy can decrease fibrinogen.*[573] Nutritional support includes garlic, coldwater fish, vitamin E, ginkgo, and bromelain. All of these substances can offset the clotting effects of fibrinogen.

Lipoprotein (a)

Lipoprotein is a small cholesterol particle that causes inflammation and can clog your blood vessels.[574, 629] Research has shown that people with elevated lipoprotein(a) have a 70% higher risk of developing heart disease over 10 years.[633]

Elevated lipoprotein(a) is inherited. Lipoprotein(a) regulates clot formation and decreases blood thinning.[575] This process is increased in diabetes and in *menopause*. Also, statin medications have been shown to increase lipoprotein(a) levels.[576]

How to lower lipoprotein(a):[634] (These are daily requirements.)

- Natural estrogen replacement
- Vitamin C (2 to 4 grams)
- Coenzyme Q-10 (120 mg)
- L-carnitine (1 to 2 grams)
- DHA (1 to 2 grams)
- Niacin (1 to 2 grams)
- L-lysine (500 to 1,000 mg)
- L-proline (500 to 1,000 mg)
- Flax seed

Dr. Stephan Sinatra in his book, *Heart Sense For Women*, has an excellent discussion of these secondary risk factors. Furthermore, he addresses the fact that the statin drugs can deplete your body of coenzyme Q-10 which may make you more vulnerable to breast cancer. These medications include Lipitor, Mevacor, Zocor, Pravachol, and others that are in a class of drugs called HMG-CoA-reductase inhibitors. Several studies have now shown that low levels of coenzyme Q-10 have been found in people with breast and cervical cancer. Therefore, if you are taking a statin drug, you should take at least 100 mg a day of coenzyme Q-10.

C-reactive Protein

Scientists believe that infection can cause heart disease. Chlamydia, herpes, and cytomegalovirus can cause inflammation in your blood vessels and cause plaque formation. Chronic gum disease and an H. pylori infection in your stomach are also causes of inflammation. C-reactive protein is an antibody-like substance that reflects the presence of a previous infection. Studies have shown that c-reactive protein can be predictive of future heart attacks even if you have a normal cholesterol level.[577, 626, 627, 628, 633]

Ways to lower C-reactive protein:[578, 634, 635]
- Exercise
- One baby aspirin a day (Ask your doctor first.)
- Essential fatty acids, EPA/DHA, fish oil (1,000 mg/day)
- Natural Cox-2 inhibitors
    - Grapeseed extract (100 to 200 mg/day)
    - Curcumin (300 to 600 mg/day)
    - Green tea (3 cups or 3 capsules/day)
- Rosemary
- Quercetin as a supplement (It is also in apples, onions, black tea.)
- Coenzyme Q-10

Nutrition

Nutrition is an important part of maximizing your HRT, preventing disease, and general treatment of menopause.

- Vitamin E helps many women by relieving hot flashes. 400 IU twice a day is a good dose.

- Boron increases estrogen production.[512] It also increases testosterone and decreases loss of calcium from your bones.[513, 514]

- A decrease in folate intake increases the incidence of breast cancer risk.[322] Folate is needed to repair your DNA.

- Fiber interrupts the estrogen pathway to decrease estrogen levels in the blood by 36%. Therefore, this can decrease your cancer risk by 54% if you are on a high fiber diet.[307]

- A deficiency in vanadium can increase progesterone. Too much vanadium can lower progesterone. Therefore, it is important to have the right amount.[523]

- Zinc is needed for making your sex hormones. It is also needed for healthy breast tissue.[524]

- Zinc may increase estrogen's bone building capability.[525]

- Zinc is needed for ovarian function and function of your adrenal glands.[526, 527]

- Zinc is part of the estrogen receptor and is needed for maximum estrogen receptor function.[155]

- Synthetic and natural estrogens have been shown to lead to a decrease in tryptophan metabolism and a decrease in B6. Supplementation is needed.[529]

- Vitamin C is needed by the ovaries to make hormones.[530]

- Vitamin A is needed to make hormones.[531]

- Vitamin E protects the adrenals and ovaries from free radical damage. Decreased vitamin E decreases hormone production.[520, 532]

Hormones and Your Skin

Your skin is a mirror of what is happening on the inside of your body.

The following are some of the causes of skin problems:
- Emotional stress
- Caffeine excess
- Saturated fats
- Refined foods and sugar
- Not enough water consumption
- Inability of your liver to detoxify
- Leaky gut syndrome
- Food allergies
- Irritating cosmetics
- Depletion of essential fatty acids
- Hormonal changes including: PMS, peri-menopause, menopause

Skin cells have estrogen receptors. As your estrogen starts declining, there is a decrease in the elastin and collagen production in your connective tissue. Estrogens increases vascularization (blood supply) to your skin and improve the structure of elastic fibers. The amount of collagen in your skin is also maintained by estrogen and decreases after menopause.[51] Estrogen furthermore, increases the water content of your skin by increasing the production of hyaluronic acid. This makes your skin soft looking and also contributes to its thickness. If you are 60-years-old and not taking estrogen your skin is only half as thick as women who do.[156] Estrogen also helps your skin look younger by maintaining the firmness. Recent studies have shown that topical estrogens, such as estriol (E3), have improved elasticity and firmness of the skin and decreased the wrinkle depth and pore size by 61% to 100%.[632] In our office we use estriol topically compounded with antioxidants by a pharmacist. We have found similar results.

A decrease in testosterone, progesterone, and growth hormone also contribute to wrinkling of your skin.

Likewise, if you want your skin to look younger, do not use petroleum based products. Mineral oil is a mixture of refined liquid hydrocarbons derived from petroleum. It is used as a stabilizing ingredient of many skin formulas.

Problems with petroleum (mineral oil) derived ingredients are:

- Petroleum based products cannot be absorbed by the skin and are foreign to its cellular structure.
- Petroleum products dry out your skin. They remove the fine coating of sebum normally found on the surface of your skin.
- Petroleum based products decrease perspiration by 40 to 60%. Perspiration is needed to allow your body to detoxify.
- Water and nutrients are blocked by petroleum products so they cannot be absorbed.

Arbonne skin care products do not contain mineral oil. For a representative in your area, call 1-800-ARBONNE.

Birth Control Pills

Affects of birth control pills on your body:

- Estrogen containing birth control pills decrease vitamins B12, folate, and B6 in your body which are needed to metabolize homocysteine. A build up of homocysteine in your body pre-disposes you to heart disease or to Alzheimer's disease. (For further explanation see the chapter on secondary risk factors for heart disease.)

- Birth control pills can deplete your body of zinc and can elevate copper levels in your system.[360]

- Women taking birth control pills have a decreased serum testosterone and DHEA.[187, 188]

- Even low-dose birth control pills contain more estrogens and progestin than is usually needed for treatment of peri-meno-pause or menopause.[474]

- Birth control pills contain progestin (synthetic progesterone). As you have seen in the chapter on progesterone, progestin use can make the symptoms of progesterone loss worse. Like-wise, progestins decrease the protective affects of estrogen on your heart.

Therefore, for all of the above reasons, birth control pills may not be the optimal HRT for peri-menopausal women.

Weight Gain in Menopause

Most women gain weight at menopause. *Weight gain is due to high levels of the wrong hormones along with losing the right hormones.*

It is the ratio of ovarian hormones that determine how much weight you gain and where you gain it:[194]

- If estradiol decreases and progesterone, testosterone, and DHEA are normal then you can gain fat around the middle.[199]

- If the ratio of estradiol to progesterone is high you gain weight around the hips.[200] Progesterone increases fat storage and decreases sensitivity to insulin.[197] *Consequently, if you only replace progesterone during menopause and you are also estrogen deficient, you can predispose yourself to weight gain and to the development of diabetes.*

- Cortisol, one of your sex hormones, facilitates the storage of body fat.[200] If cortisol increases, you store more fat, increase muscle break down, and also increase insulin resistance.

- If your cortisol level remains high your body goes into the 'flight or fight' response and you gain weight. (For a longer discussion on this subject see the chapter on cortisol.)

Other interesting facts about hormones and weight gain:

- Women who take HRT gain less weight.[56]

- Prolonged stress can decrease the function of the ovaries and consequently hormone production which can also cause a weight gain.[198]

- Obesity leads to higher levels of estrone, the estrogen associated with breast cancer.

As you can see it is very important to have your hormones in the correct ratio and amount or weight gain will be a frequent problem during and after menopause.

Surgical Menopause

One-third of women in the United States have had a hysterectomy. The average age for this operation is 35.[45]

Women who have had a partial hysterectomy (ovaries are left in) can still have a change in hormonal function. Research has now shown that about 60 to 70% of women have a decrease in hormones to menopausal levels within 3 to 4 years of surgery. For some women, progesterone levels may fall within several months of the surgery and estrogen may decline within one to two years.[237, 47] The changes in hormone levels occur because your uterine artery is cut during the hysterectomy and tied off which decreases the blood flow to your ovaries.

Other interesting facts associated with hysterectomy are:

- 40% of women who have had a hysterectomy have depression.[46]

- Surgical menopause reduces testosterone more than natural menopause.

Herbal Therapies for Menopause

Herbal supplements are wonderful to help resolve symptoms such as hot flashes and night sweats. *However, they may not be enough to maintain your bone structure, prevent heart disease, or help you maintain your memory.*

Black Cohash *(Cimicifuga racemosa)*
- Has a balancing effect on estrogen (If you have too much estrogen, black cohash lowers it and if estrogen is too low, it enhances its effects.)[42]
- Has a direct effect on the hypothalamus (brain) to decrease hot flashes
- Relaxant
- Sedative
- Anti-spasmotic
- Anti-inflammatory

Dong Quai *(Angelica archangelica)*
- Contains phytoestrogens
- Interacts with anti-coagulants

Chasteberry *(Vitex agnus castus)*
- Decreases LH and prolactin
- Raises progesterone and facilitates progesterone function
- Acts as a diuretic
- Has no known drug interactions

Salivary Testing

You should have your hormone levels measured before you begin HRT. Salivary or saliva testing is the preferred method of hormone testing for peri-menopausal women, menopausal women, and for women with PMS symptoms or other hormonal imbalances. It measures only the 'free' form of the hormones. This is important because the free hormone molecules are the only ones that can act directly on your body. Blood levels measure the amount of free and bound hormone. Saliva testing also allows for the changes of hormone levels over a number of days, as opposed to a one-time blood draw that shows levels only at the time of the test.[406, 60, 478, 479, 480, 407, 408]

Hormone levels should be repeated after you begin HRT, usually in about three months. Subsequently, tests should then be done on a routine basis depending on your own personal needs. Salivary testing will help your doctor better maintain the level of hormone replacement that is right for you.

A recently conducted study showed that 45% of women on estrogen had suboptimal levels to maintain their memory and bone structure.[468] *Researchers concluded that monitoring symptoms only was not enough.*

Therefore, repeated measurement of your hormone levels is needed in order for your doctor to optimize your HRT. Estrogen, progesterone, testosterone, cortisol, and DHEA are all hormones, like thyroid hormone, and should not be prescribed without measuring levels first and then on an ongoing basis. (See the appendix, Great Smokies Diagnostic Laboratory, for availability of salivary testing.)

Compounded Hormones

You are an individual with your own individual requirements for optimum health. Therefore, your natural HRT therapy should be made for your own individual needs. Your doctor can have a compounding pharmacist make your prescription for you and you only. Made from plant extractions, they are an exact replica of your own hormones. (For a list of compounding pharmacists see the appendix of this book.)

The key to effective hormone replacement therapy, in summary, is individuality. Fixed doses do not allow for individualized, tailor-made treatment.

Conclusion

14 keys to optimal health for peri-menopausal and menopausal women:

1. *Your hormones function as a web.* The right levels of *all* of your hormones are needed for you to achieve optimal health.

2. *Estrogen has many protective affects on your brain including maintaining your memory, decreasing the incidence of Alzheimer's disease, and lowering the rate of depression.*

3. *Estrogen is heart protective. Progestins (synthetic progesterone) stop the protective effects of estrogen on your heart. Natural progesterone is synergistic and increases the protective effects of estrogen on your heart.*

4. *It is paramount that your HRT be composed of the right kinds of estrogens: estradiol (E2) and estriol (E3).*

5. *How your body metabolizes estrogen is important.* The metabolism of estrogen via the 2-hydroxyestrone pathway is critical in lowering your risk of cancer. Have your doctor measure your urinary metabolites of 2-hydroxyestrone, 16-hydroxyestrone, and the ratio between them.

6. *Estrogen and progesterone work together in your body.* Progesterone increases your body's fat storage and decreases insulin sensitivity. Estrogen lowers your body fat, increases insulin sensitivity, and improves glucose tolerance. *Therefore, if you only replace progesterone without replacing estrogen (if you are deficient in estrogen), you may gain weight and may predispose yourself to diabetes.*

7. *Nutrients alone are not enough to prevent osteoporosis.* Estrogen, progesterone, testosterone, and DHEA are also needed.

8. *Salivary testing* of your hormone levels should be done before you begin HRT. Saliva testing is the preferred method of hormone testing. Hormone levels should be repeated after you begin HRT, and on a regular basis, to help your doctor better maintain the levels of hormones that are right for you.

9. It is very important for your body to *detoxify estrogen* completely. Have your doctor test your detoxification pathways using *Genovations* testing.

10. *Nutrition* is an important part of maximizing your HRT, preventing disease, and general treatment of menopause.

11. *Weight gain* at menopause is due, in large part, to high levels of the wrong hormones along with losing the right hormones.

12. Have your *secondary risk factors for heart disease* measured. These factors are: homocysteine, ferritin (iron), lipoprotein(a), fibrinogen, and c-reactive protein.

13. When you *stop* HRT you lose the benefits that hormones provide almost immediately.

14. Your hormone response is as unique to you as your fingerprints. *One size does not fit all.*

In summary, the answer to HRT is prescription natural hormone replacement that is customized.

Appendix I:
Compounding Pharmacies

Clark Professional Pharmacy
3075 W. Clark Rd.
Ypsilanti, MI 48197
1-800-468-0481
www.clarkpropharmacy.com

Pharmacy Solutions
5204 Jackson Rd.
Ann Arbor, MI 48103
1-734-821-8000

Health Dimensions, Inc
32985 Hamilton Ct., Suite G-200
Farmington Hills, MI 48334
1-248-489-1573

University Compounding Pharmacy
4600 Investment Dr., Suite 100
Troy, MI 48098
1-248-267-5002

Prescription Services Pharmacy
560 W. Mitchell St., Suite 200
Petosky, MI 49770
1-231-487-2147
cmrapin@northernhealth.org

College Pharmacy
3505 Austin Bluff Parkway, Suite 101
Colorado Springs, CO 80918
1-800-888-9358
www.collegepharmacy.com

Healthway Pharmacy
1008 N. Saginaw St.
St. Charles, MI 48655
1-800-742-7527

Thompson's Pharmacy and Medical
324 S. Union St.
Traverse City, MI 49684
1-800-968-4210

Madison Pharmacy Associates, Inc.
Women's Health America Group
429 Gammon Place, P.O. Box 259690
Madison, WI 53719
87-RESTORE-FU

MedQuest Pharmacy
6965 Union Park Center, Suite 100
Midvale, Utah 84047
1-888-222-2956
www.mqrx.com

Medaus Pharmacy and Compounding Center
2637 Valleydale Rd., Suite 200
Birmingham, Al 35244
1-800-526-9183
www.medaus.com
info@medaus.com

Brown's Optioncare
1015 W. Michigan Ave.
Jackson, MI 49202
1-800-253-0514

Appendix II: Laboratories

All lab testing referenced to in this book is available through:

Great Smokies Diagnostic Laboratory
63 Zillicoa St.
Asheville, NC 28801-1074
1-800-522-4762
www.gsdl.com

Appendix III: Supplements

All supplements discussed in this book are available through:

Binson's Home Health Care Centers
26819 Lawrence Ave.
Center Line, MI 48015
1-888-BINSONS
www.binsons.com

Crittenton Medical Equipment
161 S. Livernois
Rochester Hills, MI 48307
1-800-500-3808

Appendix IV: Companies That Use Pharmaceutical Grade Supplements

Supplements from the following companies are only available through your doctor, or through Binson's Home Health Care, and Crittenton Medical Equipment, which have doctors and nurses right in the store to help you with your health care needs. (See Appendix III.)

Metagenics
P.O. Box 1729
Gig Harbor, WA 98335
1-800-843-9660
www.metagenics.com

Ortho Molecular Products
3017 Business Park Drive
P.O. Box 1060
Stevens Point, WI 54481
1-800-332-2351

Vitiquest Inc./Customvite
26819 Lawrence Ave.
Center Line, MI 48015
1-888-246-7667

Designs for Health
2 North Road
East Windsor, CT 06088
1-800-847-8302
www.DesignsForHealth.com

References and Notes

1. Hammond, C., et al., "Menopause and HRT: an overview," *Obstet Gynecol* 1996; 87:2S–15S.

2. Follingstad, A., "Estriol, the forgotten estrogen?" *JAMA* 1978; 239(1):29–30.

3. Laux, M., *Natural Woman, Natural Menopause.* New York: HarperCollins, 1997, p. 20.

4. Ibid., Laux, p. 79.

5. Ibid., Laux, p. 79.

6. Stamm, W., et al., "A controlled trial of intravaginal estriol in postmenopausal women with urinary tract infections," *NEJM* 1993; 329(11):753–56.

7. Ibid., Laux, p. 8.

8. Shippen, E., *Testosterone Syndrome.* New York: M. Evans & Company Inc., 1998, p. 145.

9. Ibid., Shippen, p. 145.

10. McEwen B, et al., "Steroid and thyroid hormones modulate a changing brain," *Journal of Steroid Biochemistry and Molecular Biology* 1991; 40(1–3):1–14.

11. Henderson, V., et al., "Estrogen replacement therapy in older women. Comparisons between Alzheimer's disease cases and nondemented control subjects," *Archieves of Neurology* 1994; 51(9):896–900.

12. Paganini-Hill A., et al., "Estrogen deficiency and risk of Alzheimer's disease in women," *American Journal of Epidemiology* 1994; 140(3):256–261.

13. Tang, M., et al., "Effect of oestrogen during menopause on risk and age at onset of Alzheimer's disease," *Lancet* 1996; 348:429–432.

14. Ibid., Laux, p. 34.

15. Ibid., Laux, p. 51.

16. Lee, J., "Is natural progesterone the missing link in osteoporosis prevention and treatment?" *Medical Hypothesis* 1991; 316–18.

17. Clarkson, T., et al., "Conjugated equine estrogens alone, but not in combination with medroxyprogesterone acetate, inhibit aortic connective tissue remodeling after plasma lipid lowering in female monkeys," *Arterioscler Thromb Vasc Biol* 1998; 18(7):1164–71.

18. Ibid., Clarkson, p. 1164–71.

19. Majewska, M., et al., "Steroid hormone metabolites are barbiturate-like modulators of the GABA receptor," *Science* 1986; 232:1004.

20. Ibid., Laux, p. 119.

21. Sand, R., et al., "Exogenous androgens in postmenopausal women," *Am J. of Med* 1995; 98 (1A).

22. Sahelian, R. *DHEA, A Practical Guide.* Marina Del Ray, Calif: Be Happier Press, 1996. p.83.

23. Aksoy, I., et al., "Human live dehydroepiandosterone sulfotransferase; nature and extent of individual variation," *Clin Pharmacol Therapeutics* 1993; 54:498–506.

24. Ibid., Shippen, p. 152.

25. Barbieri, R., et al., "Cotinine and nicotine inhibit human fetal adrenal 11, beta-hydroxylase," *J Clin Endocrinol Metab* 1989; 69:1221–4.

26. Brzezinski, A., et al., "Melatonin in humans," *NEJM* 1997; 336(3):186–195.

27. Bland J., "Obesity and endocrine signaling," *Improving Intercelluar Communication in Managing Chronic Illness.* Gig Harbor Washington: Health Comm International, Inc., 1999, p. 124.

28. Ibid., Bland, p. 125.

29. Duell, P., et al., "Inhibition of LDL oxidation by melatonin requires supraphysiologic concentrations," *Clin Chem* 1998; 44(9):1931–1936.

30. Ibid., Brzezinski, p. 186–195.

31. Ibid., Bland, *Improving Intercellar Communication in Managing Chronic Illness.* p. 127.

32. Bland, J. p. 186.

33. Bunevicius, R., et al., "Effects of thyroxine as compared with thyroxine plus triiodothyroxine in patients with hypothyroidism," *NEJM* 1999; 340(6):424–429.

34. Nishiyama, S., et al., "Zinc supplementation alters thyroid hormone metabolism in disabled patients with zinc deficiency," *J. Am. Coll. Nut.* 1994; 13:62–7.

35. Meinhold, H., et al., "Effects of selenium and iodine deficiency on iodothyronine deiodinases in brain, thyroid and peripheral tissue," *JAMA* 1992; 19:8–12.

36. Berry, M., et al., "The role of selenium in thyroid hormone action," *Endocrine Rev* 1992; 13:207–20.

37. Kohrle, J., "The deiodinase family; selenoenzymes regulating thyroid hormone availability and action," *Cell Mol Life Sci* 2000; 57:1853–63.

38. Beard, J., et al., "Impaired thermoregulation and thyroid function in iron deficiency anemia," *Am. J. Clin. Nutr* 1990; 52:813–9.

39. Lenon, D., et al., "Diet and exercise training effects on resting metabolic rate," *Int. J. Obesity* 1985; 9:39–47.

40. Ibid., Laux, p. 21.

41. Sherwin, B., "Estrogen use and verbal memory in healthy post-menopausal women," *Obstetrics and Gynecology* 1994; 83(6):979–83.

42. Murray, M., *The Healing Power of Herbs.* California: Prima Publications, 1995, p. 375.

43. Ottoson, U., et al., "Subfractions of high-density lipo-protein cholesterol during estrogen replacement therapy: A comparison between progestogens and natural progesterone," *Journal of Obstetrics and Gynecology* 1985; 151:746–50.

44. Lee, J., *What Your Doctor May Not Tell You About Menopause.* New York: Warner, 1996, p. 88.

45. Cutler, W., *Hysterectomy: Before and After.* New York: Harper & Row, 1988, p. 27.

46. Vliet, E., "New insights on hormones and mood," *Menopause Management* 1993; June/July:140–46.

47. Ibid., Laux, p. 99.

48. Nabulsi, A., et al., "Association of hormone replacement therapy with various cardiovascular risk factors in post menopausal women," *NEJM* 1993; 328:1069–1075.

49. Phillips, S., et al., "Effects of estrogen on memory function in surgically menopausal women," *Psycho Neuroendocrinology* 1992; 17(5):485–495.

50. Ibid, Phillips, p. 493.

51. Ibid., Shippen p. 150.

52. Nachtigall, L. *Estrogen The Facts Can Change Your Life.* New York: HarperCollins, 1995, p. 27.

53. Michnovicz, J., et al., "Introduction of estradiol metabolism by dietary indole-3-carbinol in humans," *J. Nat Cancer Inst* 1990; 82:947–949.

54. Ibid., Nachtigall, p. 33.

55. Ibid., Nachtigall, p. 56.

56. Ibid., Nachtigall, p. 66.

57. Nestler, J., et al., "Insulin as an effector of human ovarian and adrenal steroid metabolism," *Endocrinol Met. Clincs North America* 1991; 204:807–823.

58. Bland, J., "Carbohydrate intolerance, insulin, DHEA and oxidative stress," *Nutritional Improvement of Health Outcomes—The Inflammatory Disorders* Gig Harbor, Washington:The Institute For Functional Medicine, Inc., 1997, p. 81.

59. Nestler, J., et al., "Insulin inhibits adrenal 17-20-lyase activity in man," *J. Clin Endocrinol Met* 1992; 74(2):362–367.

60. Ibid., Bland, *Nutritional Improvement of Health Outcomes—The Inflammatory Disorders* p. 81.

61. Sarrel, P., et al., "Estrogen actions in arteries, bone and brain," *Sci. Am. Med* 1994; 1:44.

62. Hays, B., "Solving the hormone replacement dilemma in perimenopause," *Functional Medicine Approaches To Endocrine Disturbances Of Aging* Gig Harbor, Washington: The Institute For Function Medicine, Inc., 2001, p.15–43.

63. Aldercreatz, J., et al., "Western diet and western diseases: some hormonal and biochemical mechanisms and associations," *Scand J. Clin Lab Invest* 1990; 50(suppl 201).

64. Woods, M., et al., "Low-fat, high fiber diet and serum estrone sulfate in premenopausal women," *Am J. Clin Nutr* 1989; 49:1179–83.

65. Schedlowski, M., et al., "Acute psychological stress increases plasma levels of cortisol, prolactin and thyroid stimulating hormone," *Life Sciences* 1992; 50:1201–5.

66. Mendleson, J., "Alcohol effects on reproductive function in women," *Psychiatr Letter* 1986; 4:35–8.

67. "Drugs that cause sexual dysfuction: an update," *The Medical Letter* 1992; 34 (Issue 876).

68. Baghurst, P., et al., "Diet, prolactin and breast cancer," *Am J. Clin Nutr* 1992; 56:943–9.

69. Ibid., Baghurst, p. 943–9.

70. Ibid., Baghurst, p. 943–9.

71. Panth, M., et al., "Effect of vitamin A supplementation on plasma progesterone and estradiol levels during pregnancy," *Int J. Vit Nutr Res* 1991; p. 61.

72. Luck, M., et al., "Ascorbic acid and fertility," *Biol Reproduc* 1995; 52:262–6.

73. Rachman, B., "Managing endocrine imbalance; autoimmune-induced thyroidopathy and chronic fatigue syndrome," *Functional Medicine Approaches to Endocrine Disturbances of Aging.* Gig Harbor, Washington: The Institute For Functional Medicine, 2001, p.226.

74. Ibid., Rachman, p. 201–234.

75. Ibid., Meinhold, p. 8–12.

76. Ibid., Tang, p. 429–432.

77. Bland, J., "Inflammation and age—related diseases: The neurological, cardiovascular, and immune connection," *Nutritional Improvement of Health Outcomes—The Inflammatory Disorders.* Gig Harbor, Washington:Health Comm., Inc., 1997, p. 276.

78. Ibid., Bland J., p. 277.

79. Ibid., Bland J., p. 278.

80. Heller, L, *The Essentials of Herbal Care Part II.* San Clemente, CA: Metagenics, Inc., 2000, p. 1144.

81. Ibid., Heller, L., p.1144.

82. Ibid., Heller, L., p.1145.

83. Ibid., Heller, L, p.1145.

84. Telang, N., et al., "Induction by estrogen metabolite 16-alpha hydroxy estrone of genotoxic damage and aberrant proliferation in mouse mammory epithelial cells," *J. Natl Cancer Inst* 1992; 84(8):634–638.

85. Bland, J., "Cellular communication and signal transduction," *Improving Intracellar Communication in Managing Chronic Illness.* Gig Harbor, Washington: The Function Medicine Institute, 1999; p.26.

86. Ibid., Bland, J. 27.

87. Ibid., Telang, p. 634–638.

88. Hankinson, S., et al., "Plasma sex steroid hormone levels and risk of breast cancer in postmenopausal women," *J. Natl Cancer Inst* 1998; 56(2):S20–S21.

89. Ibid., Bland, *Intracellular Communication in Managing Chronic Illness*, p. 118.

90. Regelson, W., et al., "Hormonal intervention: buffer hormones or state dependency. The role of dehydroepiandrosterone (DHEA), thyroid hormone, estrogen, and hypophysectomy in aging," *Ann NY Acad Sci* 1988; 521:260–273.

91. Paech, K., et al., "Differential ligand activation of estrogen receptors ER a and ER b at AP1 sties," *Science* 1997; 277(5331):1508–1510.

92. Zhu, B., et al., "Functional role of estrogen metabolism in target cells: review and perspectives," *Carcinogenesis* 1998; (1):1–27.

93. Nagata, C., et al., "Decreased serum estradiol concentration associated with high dietary intake of soy products in pre-menopausal Japanese women," *Nutr Cancer* 1997; 29(3):228–233.

94. Sherwin, B., et al., "Estrogen and cognitive functioning in surgi-cally menopausal women," *Ann NY Acad Sci* 1990; 592:474–475.

95. Xu, H., et al., "Estrogen reduces neuronal generation of Alzheimer's B-amyloid peptides," *Nature Med* 1998; 4(4):447–451.

96. Ibid., Bland, *Intracellular Com-munication in Managing Chronic Illness*, p. 127.

97. Ballinger, S., et al., "Stress as a factor in lowered estrogen levels in the early menopause," *Ann NY Acad Sci* 1990; 592:95–113.

98. Pansini, F., et al., "Control of carbohydrate metabolism in menopausal women receiving transdermal estrogen therapy," *Ann NY Acad Sci* 1990; 592:460–462.

99. Ibid., Bland., *Intracellular Communication in Managing Chronic Illness*, p. 128.

100. Rouzier, N., "Estrogen and progesterone replacement," *Longevity and Preventive Medicine Symposium.* 2002, p.8.

101. Rouzier, N., "Thyroid replace-ment therapy," *Longevity and Preventive Medicine Symposium.* 2002, p.2.

102. Ibid., Rouzier p. 3.

103. Ibid., Rouzier p. 4.

104. Hale, A., et al., "Subclinical hypothyroidism is an indepen-dent risk factor for atherosclerosis and MI in elderly women: The Rotterdam study," *Ann Inter Med* 2000; 132:270–278.

105. Bunevicius, R., et al., "Effects of thyroxine as compared with thyroxine plus triiodothyroxine in patients with hypothyroidism," *NEJM* 1999; Feb. 11:424.

106. Ibid., Rouzier, p. 16.

107. Ibid., Rouzier, p. 12.

108. Ibid., Rouzier, p. 13.

109. Ibid., Rouzier, p. 14.

110. Ibid., Rouzier, p. 13.

111. Colditz, G., et al., "Use of estrogen plus progestin is associated with greater increase in brest cancer risk than estrogen alone," *Am J. Epidemiol* 1998; 147(suppl):64S.

112. Schairer, C., et al., "Menopausal estrogen and estrogen-progestin replacement therapy and breast cancer risk," *JAMA* 2000; 283:485–491.

113. Hanley, J., "Female Empower-ment in the decisions from PMS to menopause," *Functional Medicine Approaches to Endocrine Disturbances of Aging.* Gig Harbor, Washington:The Func-tional medicine Institute, 2001; p. 12

114. Sowers, M., "A prospective study of bone mineral content and fracture in communities with differential fluoride exposure," *Am J. Epidemiol* 1991; 133(7):649–60.

115. Bland, J. "Introduction to neuroendocrine disorders," *Functional Medicine Approaches to Endocrine Disturbances of Aging.* Gig Harbor, Washington: The Functional Medicine Institute, 2001; p. 57.

116. van Baal, W., et al., "Cardiovascular disease risk and hormone replacement therapy(HRT). A review based on randomized, controlled studies in postmenopausal women," *Curr Med Chem* 2000; 7(5):499–517.

117. Barnebei, V., et al., "Plasma homocysteine in women taking hormone replacement therapy: the post menopausal estrogen/progestin interventions (PEPI) trial," *J. Women's Health Gend Based Med* 1999; 8(9):1167–1172.

118. Brown, C., et al., "The C677T methylenetetrahydrofolate reductase polymorphism influences the homocysteine-lowering effect of hormone replacement therapy," *Mol Genet Metab* 1999; 67(1):43–48.

119. Stoney C., et al., " Plasma homocysteine levels increase in women during psychological stress," *Life Sci* 1999; 64(25):2359–2365.

120. DeCree, C., et al., "Influence of exercise and menstrual cycle phase on plasma homocysteine levels in young women—prospective study," *Scand J. Med Sci Sports* 1999; 9(5):272–278.

121. Ibid., Bland, *Functional Medicine Approaches to Endocrine Disturbances of Aging*, p. 61.

122. Hak A., et al., "Increased plasma homocystine after menopause," *Atherosclerosis* 2000; 149(1):163–168.

123. Ibid., van Baal, p. 499–517.

124. Nourhashemi, F., et al., "Alzheimer's disease: protective factors," *Am J.Clin Nutr* 2000; 71(2):643S–649S.

125. Carmel, R., et al., "Hormone replacement therapy and cobalamin status in elderly women," *Am J. Clin Nutr* 1996: 64(6):856–859.

126. Ibid., Bland, *Functional Medicine Approaches to Endocrine Disturbances of Aging*, p. 62

127. Drouva S., et al., "Estradiol activates methylating enzyme(s) involved in the conversion of phosphatidyl-ethanolamine to phosphatidlylcholine in rat pituitary membranes," *Endocrinol* 1986; (1996):2611–2622.

128. Molloy, A., et al., "Thermolabile variant of 5,10-methylenetetrahydrofolate reductase associated with low red-cell folates: implications for folate intake recommendations," *Lancet* 1997; 349:1591–1593.

129. Ibid., Bland, *Functional Medicine Approaches to Endocrine Disturbances of Aging*, p. 68.

130. Bradlow, H., et al., "Selective induction of cytochrome P450 enzymes in the prevention of breast cancer," *The New Biology of Steroid Hormones* Serono Symposium 1991; 74:125–144.

131. Michnovicz, J., et al., Dietary cytochrome P450 modifiers in the control of estrogen metabolism. Food phytochemicals for cancer prevention," *American Chem Society* 1994; 282–293.

132. Bradlow, H., et al., Indole-3-carbinol: A novel approach to breast cancer prevention," *First International on Cancer Prevention Proceedings of the NY Academy of Sciences* 1996; 768:180–200.

133. Bradlow, H., et al., "Dietary modulation of estrogen metabolism: a novel approach to cancer chemoprevention," _Fundamentals of Cancer Prevention_ 1996; p. 41–44.

134. Bradlow, H., et al., "Multifunctional aspects of the action of indole-3-carbinol as a anti-tumor agent," _NY Acad Sci_ 1999; 889:204–213.

135. Telang, N., et al., "Cell cycle regulation, apoptosis and estradiol biotransformation: novel endpoint biomarkers for human breast cancer prevention," _J. Clin Ligand Assay_, 2000.

136. Michnovicz, J., et al., "Induction of estradiol metabolism by dietary indole-3-carbinol in humans," _J. Natl Cancer Inst_ 1990; 50:947–950.

137. Jellinck, P., et al., "Influences of indole-3-carbinol on the hepatic microsomal formation of catechol estrogen," _Steroid_ 1991; 56:446–450.

138. Michnovicz, J., et al., "Altered estrogen metabolism and excretion in humans following consumption of indole-3-carbinol," _Nutr Cancer_ 1991; 16:59–66.

139. Osborne, M., et al., "Increases in the extent of etradiol 16-alpha-hydroxylation in human breast tissue: a potential biomarkers of breast cancer risk," _J. Natl Cancer Inst_ 1993; 85:1917–1920.

140. Ibid., Bland, _Functional Medicine Approaches to Endocrine Disturbances of Aging_, p. 121.

141. Ibid., Bland, p. 121.

142. Ibid., Bland, p. 121.

143. Ibid., Bland, p. 121.

144. Ibid., Schairer, p. 485–491.

145. Clemors, M., et al., "Estrogen and the risk of breast cancer," _NEJM_ 2001; 344:276–285.

146. Yaffe, K., et al., "Cognitive decline in women in relation to non-protein-bound oestradiol concentrations," _Lancet_ 2000; 356:708–712.

147. Mulnard, R., et al., "Estrogen replacement therapy for treatment of mild to moderate Alzheimer's disease," _JAMA_ 2000; 283:1007–15.

148. Baulieu, E., et al., "Progesterone as a neuroactive neurosteroid, with special references to the effect of progesterone on myelination," _Hum Reprod_ 2000; Suppl:1–13.

149. Poeggeler, B., et al., "Melatonin—a highly potent endogenous radical scavenger and electron donor: new aspects of the oxidation chemistry of this indole accessed in vitro," _Ann NY Acad Sci_ 1994; 738:419–421.

150. Ibid., Barbier, p. 1221–1224.

151. Yeh, J., et al., "Nicotine and cotinine inhibit rat testes androgen biosynthesis in vitro," _J. Steroid Biochem_ 1989; 33(4A):627–630.

152. Michnovicz J., et al., "Environmental modulation of oestrogen metabolism in humans," _Int'l Clin Nutr Rev_ 1987: 7(4):169–173.

153. Visser, T., et al., "Role of sulfation in thyroid hormone metabolism," _Chem Biol Interactions_ 1994; 92:293–303.

154. Aksoy, I., et al., "Human liver dehydroepiandrosterone sulfatransferase: nature and extent of individual variation,"

Clin Pharmacol Therapeutics 1993; 54(5):498–506.

155. Walsh, C., et al., "Zinc: health effects and research priorities for the 1990s," *Envir Health Perspect* 1994; 102, (suppl2):5–46.

156. Ibid., Shippen, p. 150.

157. Ushiroyama, T., et al., "Efficacy of ipriflavone and 1-alpha vitamin D therapy for the cessation of vertebral bone loss," *Int J. Gynecol Obstetrics* 1995; 48:283–288.

158. Windsor, A., et al., "The effect of whole-bone extract on 47C and absorption in the elderly," *Age Ageing* 1973; 2:230–234.

159. Agnusdei, D., et al., "Metabolic and clinical effects of ipriflavone in established postmenopausal osteoporosis," *Drugs Exptl Clin Res* 1989; XV(2):97–104.

160. Roberts, E., et al., "Pregnenolone—from Selye to Alzheimer's and a model of the pregnenolone sulfate binding site on the GABA receptor," *Biochemical Pharmacology* 1995; vol 49, no.1, p. 1–16.

161. Ibid., Bland, *Functional Medicine Approaches to Endocrine Disturbances of Aging*, p. 65.

162. Lee, J., *What Your Doctor May Not Tell You About Premenopause.* New York: Warner Books, 1999, p. 4.

163. Ibid., Bland, *Funcitonal Medicine Approaches to Endocrine Disturbances of Aging*, p. 65.

164. Ibid., Bland, p. 66.

165. Ibid., Bland, p. 70.

166. Ibid., Bland, p. 71.

167. Ibid., Bland, p. 71.

168. Ibid., Bland, p. 71.

169. Ibid., Bland, p. 71.

170. Ibid., Bland, p. 73.

171. Ibid., Bland, p. 74.

172. Kaaks, R., et al., "Nutrition, hormones and breast cancer: is insulin the missing link?" *Cancer Causes Control* 1996; 7:605–625.

173. Ibid., Bland, *Functional Medicine Approaches to Endocrine Disturbances of Aging*, p. 73.

174. Greendale, G., et al., "The menoapuse transition," *Endocrinol Metab Clin NA* 1997; 26(2):261–277.

175. The Postmenopausal Estrogen/Progestin Interventions (PEPI) trial: *National Heart, Lung, and Blood Institute*, Nov 17, 1994; 1–4.

176. Ibid., (PEPI), p. 1–4.

177. Ibid., Bland, *Functional Medicine Approaches to Endocrine Disturbance of Aging*, p. 80.

178. Writing group for the PEPI, "Effect of hormone therapy on bone mineral density: results from the postmenopausal estrogen/progestin interventions (PEPI) trial," *JAMA* 1996; 276(17):1389–1396.

179. Ibid., Bland, *Functional Medicine Approaches to Endocrine Disturbances of Aging*, p. 80.

180. Ross, R., et al., "Effect of hormone replacement therapy on breast cancer risk: estrogen versus estrogen plus progestin," J. Natl Cancer Inst 1992; (4):328–332.

181. Ibid., Schairer, p. 485–491.

182. Ibid., Bland, Functional Medicine Approaches to Endocrine Disturbances of Aging, p. 83.

183. Vliet, E, *Women Weight and Hormones*, New York: M. Evans & Company , 2001; p. 25.

184. Ibid., Nachtigall, p. 127.

185. Ibid., Nachtigall, p. 156.

186. Brownstein, D., *The Miracle of Natural Hormones*. West Bloomfield, Michigan: Medical Alternatives Press, 1998, p. 11.

187. Ibid., Browstein, p. 54.

188. Coenen, C., et al., "Changes in androgens during treatment with four low-dose contraceptives," *Contraception* 1996; 53(3):171–6.

189. Prior, J., et al., "Progesterone as a bone trophic hormone," *Endocrine Reviews* 1990; 11:386–398.

190. *Nutrition and Healing Newsletter,* 1995; Vol 11, No. 12.

191. Hardeland R., et al., "The significance of the metabolism of the neurohormone melatonin: antioxidative protection and formation of bioactive substances," *Neuroscience and Biobehavioral Reviews* 1993; 17:347–57.

192. Ibid., Vliet, p. 50.

193. Ibid., Vliet, p. 31.

194. Ibid., Vliet, p. 35.

195. Rosano, G., et al., "Syndrome X in women is associated with estrogen deficiency," *Eur Heart J.* 1995; 16:610–14.

196. Ibid., Vliet, p. 39.

197. Ibid., Vliet, p. 40.

198. Ibid., Vliet, p. 40.

199. Ibid., Vliet, p. 40.

200. Ibid., Vliet, p. 39.

201. Ibid., Vliet, p. 45.

202. Ibid., Vliet, p. 45.

203. Ibid., Vliet, p. 45.

204. Ibid., Vliet, p. 45.

205. Ibid., Vliet, p. 58.

206. Ibid., Vliet, p. 49.

207. Ibid., Vliet, p. 49.

208. Ibid., Vliet, p. 49.

209. Ibid., Vliet, p. 69.

210. Ibid., Vliet, p. 81.

211. Ibid., Vliet, p. 81.

212. Ibid., Vliet, p. 81.

213. Ibid., Vliet, p. 84.

214. Aloia, J., et al., "Relationship of menopause to skeletal and muscle mass," *Am J. Clin Nut* 1991: 53:1378–83.

215. Ibid., Vliet, p. 85.

216. Fonseea, E., et al., "Increased serum levels of growth hormone and insulin-like growth factor—associated with simultaneous decrease of circulating insulin in postmenopausal women receiving hormone replacement therapy," *Menoapuse J. North Amer Men Soc* 1999; 6-1:56–60.

217. Nike, E., et al., "Estrogens as antioxidants," *Methods Enczymol* 1990; 186:330.

218. Ibid., Vliet, p. 88.

219. Ibid., Vliet, p. 88.

220. Ibid., Vliet, p. 88.

221. Ibid., Vliet, p. 93.

222. Ibid., Vliet, p. 95.

223. Ibid., Vliet, p. 96.

224. Ibid., Vliet, p. 97.

225. Ibid., Vliet, p. 97.

226. Ibid., Vliet, p. 97.

227. Ibid., Vliet, p. 98.

228. Ibid., Vliet, p. 98.

229. Ibid., Vliet, p. 99.

230. Ibid., Vliet, p. 99.

231. Ibid., Vliet, p. 100.

232. Ibid., Vliet, p. 100.

233. Ibid., Vliet, p. 100.

234. Kalkoff, R., et al., "Metabolic effects of progesterone," *J. Obstect Gynecol* 1982; 142–6:735–738.

235. Bhatia, S., et al., "Progesterone Suppression of the plasma growth hormone response," *J. Clin Endocrinol Metab* 1972; 35:364–369.

236. DeLignieres, B., et al., "Influence of route of administration in progesterone metabolism," *Maturitas* 1995; 21:251–257.

237. Ibid., Vliet, p. 107.

238. Ibid, Bland, *Functional Medicine Approaches to Endocrine Disturbances of Aging*, p. 84.

239. Ibid., Bland, p. 88.

240. Ibid., Bland, p. 91.

241. Fleisher, M., et al., "Estrogen metabolite ratios as biomarkers of hormonally related breast cancer risk," *Clinc Chem* 1996; 42(6):S261.

242. Bradlow, H., et al., "2-hydroxy estone: the 'good' estrogen," *J. Endocrinol* 1996; 150:S59–S265.

243. Kabat, E., et al., "Urinary estrogen metabolites and breast cancer, a case-control study," *Cancer Epidemiol Biomarkers Prev* 1997; 6:505–509.

244. Melilahn, E., et al., "Do urinary oestrogen metabolites predict breast cancer? Guernsey III cohort follow-up," *Br J. Cancer* 1998; 78(9):1250–1255.

245. Davis, D., et al., "Can environmental estrogens cause breast cancer?" *Scientific American* 1995; 273:166–170, 172.

246. Bradlow, H., et al., "Effects of pesticides on the ratio of 16-alpha:2-hydroxyestone: a biologic marker of breast cancer risk," *Environ Health Prospect* 1995; 103 (suppl 17):147–150.

247. Ibid., Bland., *Functional Medicine Approaches to Endocrine Disturbances of Aging*, p. 113.

248. Ibid., Vliet, p. 108.

249. Ibid., Vliet, p. 109.

250. Ibid., Vliet, p. 110.

251. Ibid., Vliet, p. 110.

252. Ibid., Vliet, p. 127.

253. Divi, R., et al., "Anti-thyroid isoflavones from soybean: isolation, characterization, and mechanism of action," Biochem Pharmacol 1997; 54:10, 1087–96.

254. Ibid., Vliet, p. 128.

255. Ibid., Vliet, p. 129.

256. Ibid., Vliet, p. 129.

257. Ibid., Vliet, p. 132.

258. Ibid., Vliet, p. 134.

259. Ibid., Vliet, p. 132.

260. Ibid., Vliet, p. 140.

261. Ibid., Vliet, p. 140.

262. Ibid., Vliet, p. 140.

263. Ibid., Vliet, p. 145.

264. Hedaya, R., et al., "The role of functional medicine in the treatment of depressive disorders," *Disorders of the Brain: Emerging Therapies in Complex Neurologic and Psychiatric Conditions.* Gig Harbor, Washington: Institute For Functional Medicine, 2002; p. 103.

265. Hollowell, J., et al., "Serum TSH, T4 and thyroid antibodies in the US population (1988–1994): National Health and Nutrition Examination Survey (NHANES III)," *J. Clin Endocrinol* Met 2002; 87(2):489–99.

266. Hays, B., "Estrogen and depression," *Disorders of the Brain: Emerging Therapies in Complex Neurologic and Psychiatric Conditions.* Gig Harbor, Washington: Institute For Functional Medicine, Inc., 2002; p. 269–270.

267. Bethea, C., et al., "Ovarian steroids and seratonin neural function," *Molecular Neurobiology* 1998; 18:87–123.

268. Ibid., Hays, p. 280.

269. Melton, L., et al., "Progestins reverse some of the effects of estrogen,: *TEM* 2000; 11(2):69–71.

270. Halbreich, U., et al., *CNS Drugs*, 2001:15(10):797–817.

271. Ibid., Bradlow, *Environ Health Perspec* p. 147–150.

272. Bland, J., "Disorders of intercellular mediators and messengers from a function medicine perspective," *Disorders of Intercellular Mediators and Messengers.* Gig Harbor, Washington, Institute For Functional Medicine, Inc., 1999; p. 21.

273. Tan, D., et al., "Melatonin: a potent endogeneous hydroxyl radical scavenger," *Endocrine J.* 1993; 1:57–60.

274. Lieberman, S., *The Real Vitamin and Mineral Book.* New York: Avery Publishing, 1997; p. 216.

275. Ibid., Lieberman, p. 216.

276. Ibid., Lieberman, p. 216.

277. Ibid., Lieberman, p. 216.

278. Ibid., Lieberman, p. 216.

279. Ibid., Lieberman, p. 216.

280. Ibid., Lieberman, p. 217.

281. Ibid., Lieberman, p. 217.

282. Baum, J., et al., "Long-term intake of soy protein improves blood lipid profile and increases mononuclear cell low-density-lipoprotein receptor messenger RNA in hypercholesterolemia, post-menopausal women," *Am J. Clin Nutr* 1998; 68(3):545–551.

283. Ibid., Lieberman, p. 220.

284. McCully, K., "Homocysteine and the heart revolution," *Disorders of Intercellular Mediators and Messengers, Their Relationship to Functional Illness,* Gig Harbor, Washington: The Functional Medicine Institute, 1999; p.87.

285. Ibid., McCully, p. 87.

286. Ibid., McCully, p. 87.

287. Ibid., McCully, p. 87.

288. Ibid., Liberman, p. 201.

289. Ibid., Liberman, p. 201.

290. Ibid., Liberman, p. 200.

291. Ibid., Liberman, p. 199.

292. *American Journal of Med* 1993; 95 (suppl 5A):69–74.

293. Lemon, H., et al., "Pathophysiologic considerations in the treatment of menopausal symptoms with estrogens: the role of estriol in the prevention of mammary carcinoma," *ACTA Endocrinol* 1980; 233 (suppl):17–27.

294. Arnot, B., *The Breast Cancer Prevention Diet*, New York:Little Brown and Company, 1998; p. 35

295. Ibid., Arnot, p. 34.

296. Ibid., Arnot, p. 38.

297. Ibid., Arnot, p. 38.

298. Ibid., Arnot, p. 82.

299. Ibid., Arnot, p. 92.

300. Ibid., Arnot, p. 92.

301. Ibid., Arnot, p. 93.

302. Ibid., Arnot, p. 95.

303. Ibid., Arnot, p. 95

304. Ibid., Arnot, p. 96.

305. Ibid., Arnot, p. 60.

306. Ibid., Arnot, p. 61.

307. Ibid., Arnot, p. 113.

308. Ibid., Arnot, p. 154.

309. Warga, C, *Menopause and the Mind*, New York: Simon and Schuster, 1999; p. XVII

310. Ibid., Warga, p. 87

311. Ibid., Warga, p. 92.

312. Ibid., Warga, p. 94

313. Ibid., Warga, p. 101.

314. Kimura, D., et al., "Estrogen replacement therapy may protect against intellectual decline in postmenopausal woman," *Hormones and Behavior*, 1995; 29:312–321.

315. Ibid., Warga, p. 234.

316. Ibid., Warga, p. 236.

317. Ibid., Warga, p. 284.

318. Writing Group for the Women's Health Initiative Investigators, "Risk and benefits of estrogen plus progestin in healthy post-menopausal women," *JAMA* 2002; 288:321–333.

319. *Mayo Clinic Women's Health Source*, Sept 2002; p. 3.

320. Grady, E., et al., "Cardiovascular disease outcomes during 6.8 years of hormone therapy," *JAMA* 2002; 288(1)49–57.

321. Muti., P., et al., "Estrogen metabolism and risk of breast cancer; a prospective study of the 2:16 alpha hydroxy estrogen ratio in premenopausal and postmenopausal women," *Epidemiology* 2000; 11:635–40.

322. Shrubsole, M., et al., "Dietary folate intake and breast cancer risk results form the Shanghai Breast Cancer Study," *Cancer Res* 2001; 61(19):7136–41.

323. Purobit, A., et al., "The role of cytokines in regulating estrogen synthesis implications for the etiology of breast cancer," *Breast Cancer Res* 2002; 4(2):65–9.

324. Yudkin, J., et al., "Inflammatin, obesity, stress and carciovascular disease is interleukin-6 the link?" *Atherosclerosis* 2000; 148(2):209–14.

325. Heinrich, P., et al., "Interleukin-6 and the acute phase response," *Biochem J.* 1990; 265:621–636.

326. Ibid., Writing Group For The Women's Health Initiative, p. 321–333.

327. Rosendaal, F., et al., "Hormonal replacement therapy, prothrombotic mutations and the risk of venous thrombosis," Br J. *Hematol* 2002; 116(4):851–4.

328. Psaty, B., et al., "Hormone replacement therapy, prothrombotic mutations, and the risk of incident nonfatal MI in postmenopausal women," *JAMA* 2001; 285(7):906–13.

329. Kurabayashi, T., et al., "Association of vitamin D and estrogen receptor gene polymorphism with the effect of hormone replacement therapy on bone mineral density in Japanese women," *Am J. Obstet Gynecol* 1999; 180(5):1115–20.

330. Ibid., Meilahn, p. 1250–1255.

331. Loscaizo, J., et al., "Lipoprotein (a): a unique risk factor for atherothrombotic disease," *Arterlosclerosis* 1990; 10(5):672–9.

332. Espeland, M., et al., "Effect of postmenopausal hormone therapy on lipoprotein (a) concentration PEPI investigators, postmenopausal estrogen/progestin interventions," *Circulation* 1998; 97(10):979–86.

333. Barnabei, V., et al., "Plasma homocysteine in women taking hormone replacement therapy; the postmenopausal estrogen/progestin intervention (PEPI) trial," *J. Women's Health Gen Based Med* 1999; 8(9):1167–72.

334. Wilkin, T., et al., "Changing perceptions in osteoporosis," *Br Med J.* 1999; 318:862–5.

335. Flore, C., et al., "Response of biochemical markers of bone turnover to estrogen treatment in post-menopausal women: evidence against an early anabolic effect on bone formation," *J. Endocrinol Invest* 2001; 24:423–9.

336. Hesley, R., et al., "Monitoring estrogen replacement therapy and identifying rapid bone loses with an immunoessay for deoxypyridinoline," Osteoporosis Int 1998; 8(2):159–64.

337. Dupont, E., et al., "The prognostic value of altered estrogen metabolism in breast cancer," *Annuals of Surgical Oncology* 2000; 7(1): supplement.

338. Dupont, E., et al., "Prognostic value of altered estrogen metabolism in breast cancer patients on premarin," Poster 1694 37th Am Soc of Clinical Oncology Meeting, May 2001.

339. Bradlow, H., et al., "Long-term responses of woman to indole-3-carbinol or a high fiber diet," *Cancer Epidemology, Biomarkers and* Prevention 1994; vol 3:591–595.

340. Fowke, J., et al., "Brassica vegetable consumpton shift's estrogen metabolism in healthy postmenopausal women," *Cancer Epidemology Biomarkers and Prevention* 2000; Vol 9:773–779.

341. Fishman, J., et al., "Increased estrogen 16-alpha hydroxylase activity in women with breast and endometrial cancer," *J. Steroid Biochem* 1984; Apr 20(4B):1077–81.

342. Wong, G., et al., "Dose-ranging study of indole-3- carbinol for breast cancer prevention," *Journal of Cellular Biochemistry* 1997; Suppl 28/29:1111–1161.

343. Bradlow, H., et al., "Estrogen metabolism and risk of breast cancer; a prospective study of the 2:16 alpha hydroxy estrone ratio in premenopausal and postmenopausal women," *Epidemiology* 2000; 11(6):635–40.

344. Heaad, K., "Estriol: safety and efficacy," Alern Med Rev 1998; 3(2):101–13.

345. Meilahn, E., "Do urinary oestrogen metabolites predict breast cancer?" *Guersey III Cohort Follow-up* 1998; 78(9): 1250–1255.

346. Fahracus, L., et al., "Norgestrel and progesterone have difference influences on plasma lipoproteins," *Eur J. Clin Invest* 1983;13:447–53.

347. Ottson, U., et al., "Oral progesterone and estrogen/progestogen therapy," *ACTA Ostet Gynecol Scand* 1984; 27 (suppl): 1–37.

348. Ottson, U., et al., "Subfractions of high-density lipoprotein cholesterol during estrogen replacement therapy a comparison between progetogens and natural progesterone," *Am J. Obstet Gynecol* 1985; 151:746–50.

349. Simpkins, J., et al., "Estrogen may be useful therapy for Alzheimer's disease and other neurodegenerative diseases," *Am J. Med* 1997; 103(3A):19S–23S.

350. Ibid., Tang, p. 429–432.

351. Ohkura, T., et al. "Low-dose estrogen replacement for Alzheimer's disease in women," *J. North Am Menopause Soc* 1994; 1:125–130.

352. Manvais-Jarvis, P., et al., "Progesterone and progestins: a general overview," *Progesterone and Progestins*, New York: Rave Press, 1983; p. 1–16.

353. Ottosson, U., et al., "Oral progesterone and estrogen/progestogen therapy, effects of natural and synthetic hormones on subfractions of HDL cholesterol and liver proteins," *ACTA Obstet Gynecol Scand* 1984; (suppl), 127:1–37.

354. Henderson, B., et al., "Estrogen replacement therapy and protection form acute MI," *Am J. Obstet Gynecol* 1988; 159:312–7.

355. Lemon, H., et al., Estriol prevention of mammary carcinoma induced by 7, 12-dimethylbenzanthracene and procarbazine," *Cancer Res* 1975; 35:1341–1352.

356. Lemon, H., et al, "Reduced estriol excretion in patients with breast cancer prior to endocrine therapy," *JAMA* 1966; 196(13):1129–36.

357. Lauritzen, C., et al., "Results of a 5 years prospective study of estriol succinate treatment in patients with climacteric complaints," *Horm Metabol Res* 1987; 19:579–584.

358. Yanick, P., *Prohormone Nutrition*, Montclair, NJ:Longevity Institute International, 1998; p. 358.

359. Ibid., Yanick, p. 41.

360. Ibid., Yanick, p. 43.

361. Michnovicz, J., et al., "Induction of estradiol metabolism by dietary indole-3-carbinol in humans," *J. Natl Cancer Inst* 1990; 82:947–949.

362. Schneider, J., et al., "Effects of obesity on estradiol metabolism: decreased formation of nonuterotropic metabolites," *J. Clin. Endocrinol Metab* 1983; 56:973–978.

363. Ballard-Barbask, R., et al., "Body weight: estimation of risk of breast and endometrial cancers," *Am J. Clin Nutr* 1996; 63: 437S–441S.

364. Vermeulen, A., et al., "Sex hormone concentrations in postmenopausal women, relation to obesity, fat mass, age and years postmenopause," *Clinic Endo* 1978; 9:59–66.

365. Longscope, C., et al., "Androgen and estrogen metabolism: relationship to obesity," *Metabolism* 1986; 35:235–2137.

366. Potischman, N., et al., "Case-control study of endogenous steroid hormones and endometrial cancer," *J. Natl Cancer Inst* 1996; 88:1127–1135.

367. Michnovicz, J., et al., "Increased estrogen 2-OH in obese women using oral indole-3-carbinol," *International Journal of Obesity* 1998; 22:227–229.

368. Michnovicz, J., et al., "Changes in levels of urinary estrogen metabolites after oral indole-3-carbinol treatment in humans," *J. Natl Canc Inst* 1997; 89(10):718–23.

369. Michnovicz, J., et al., "Induction of estradiol metabolism by dietary indole-3-carbinol in humans," *J. Natl Canc Inst* 1990; 82:947–9.

370. Fishman, J., et al., "Biological properties of 16-alpha hydroxy estrone: implications in estrogen physiology and pathophysiology," *J. Clin Endocrinol Metab* 1980; 51:611–615.

371. Zhu, B., et al., "Is 2-methoxyestradiol an endogenous estrogen metabolite that inhibits mammary carcinogenesis?" *Cancer Res* 1998; 58:2269–2277.

372. Martucci, C., et al., "P450 enzymes of estrogen metabolism," *Pharmacol Ther* 1993; 57:237–257.

373. Ursin, G., et al., "Urinary 2-hydroxy estrone/16 alpha hydroxy esrone ratio; risk of breast cancer in postmenopausal women," *J. Natl Canc Inst*, 1999; 91:1067–1072.

374. De Cree, C., et al., "4-hydroxycatecholestrogen metabolism responses to exercise and training: possible implications for menstrual cycle irregularities and breast cancer," *Fertil Steril* 1997; 67:505–516.

375. Anderson, K., "The influence of dietary protein and carbohydrate on the principal oxidative biotransformation of estradiol in normal subjects," *J. Clin Endocrinol Metabolism* 1984; 59:103–107.

376. Lu, L., "Increased urinary excretion of 2-hydroxy estrone but not 16-alpha hydroxy estrone in premenopausal women during a soy diet containing isoflavones," *Cancer Research* 2000; 60:1299–1305.

377. Haggans, C., et al., "Effect of flax seed consumption on urinary estrogen metabolites in post-menopausal women," *Nutrition and Cancer*, 1999; 33(2):188–195.

378. Bush, t., et al., "Preserving cardiovascular benefits of hormone replacement therapy," *Journal of Reproductive Med* 2000; 45(3)suppl:259–73.

379. Fishman, J., et al., "The role of estrogen in mammary carcinogenesis," *Ann NY Acad Sci* 1995; 768:91–100.

380. Ibid., Fishman, p. 611–615.

381. Fishman, J., et al., "Increased estrogen 16-alpha hydroxylase activity in women with breast

and endometrial cancer," *J. Steroid Biochem* 1984; 20:1077–1081.

382. Bradlow, H., et al., "2-hydroxy estrone" the 'good' estrogen," *J. Endocrinol* 1996; 150 (suppl):S259–S265.

383. Kabut, G., et al., "Urinary estrogen metabolites and breast cancer: a case-control study," *Cancer Epidemiol Biomarkers Prev* 1997; 6:505–509.

384. Anderson, K., et al., "The influence of dietary protein and carbohydrate on the principal oxidative biotransformations of estradiol in normal subjects," *J. Clin Endocr Metab* 1984; 59:103–107.

385. Longcope, C., et al., "The effect of a low fat diet on estrogen metabolism," *J. Clin Endocrinol Met* 1987; 64:1246–1250.

386. Kall, M., et al., "Effects of dietary broccoli on human in vivo drug metabolizing-enzymes: eval of caffeine, oestrone and chlorzoxazone metabolism," *Carcinogenesis* 1996; 17:793–799.

387. Ibid., Bradlow, *Cancer Epidemiol Biomarkers Prev*, p. 591–595.

388. Ibid., Michnovicz, *J. Nat Canc Instit*, p. 718–723.

389. Osborne, M., et al., "Omega 3 fatty acids; modulation of estrogen metabolism and potential for breast cancer prevention," *Cancer Invest* 1988; 8:629–631.

390. Stefanick, M., et al., "Estrogen, progestogens and cardiovascular risk: review of PEPPI trial," *J. Repro Med* 1999; 44(2suppl):221–6.

391. Gerhard, M., et al., "Estradiol therapy combined with progesterone; endothelium-dependent vasodilation in postmenopausal women," *Circulation* 1998; 98(12);1158–63.

392. Paganini-Hill, A., et al., "Estrogen replacement therapy and risk of Alzheimer's disease," *Arch Intern Med* 1996; 156:2213–2217.

393. Paganini-Hill, A., et al., "Estrogen deficiency and risk of Alzheimer's disease in women," *Am J. Epidemiol* 1994;140:256–261.

394. Tzay-Shing, Y., et al., "Efficacy and safety of estriol replacement therapy for climacteric women," *Chin Med J.* (Taipei) 1995; 55:386–91.

395. Tzingourius, V., et al., "Estriol in the management of the menopause," *JAMA* 1978; 239:1638–1641.

396. Michnovicz, J. et al., "Cimetidine inhibits catechol estrogen metabolism in women," *Metabolism* 1991; 40:170–74.

397. Ibid., Yanick, p. 57.

398. Haggins, C., et al., "Effect of flaxseed consumption in postmenopausal women," *Nut Cancer* 1999; 33(2):188–15.

399. Dwivedi, C., et al., "Effect of calcium glucurate on B-glucuronidase activity and glucarate content of certain vegetables and fruits," *Biochem Med Metab Biol* 1990; 43:83–92.

400. van Baal W., et al., "Cardiovascular disease risk and hormone replacement therapy (HRT); a review based on randomized, controlled studies in postmeno-

pausal woman," *Curr Med Chem* 2000; 5:499–517.

401. Barnebei, V., et al., "Plasma homocysteine in women taking hormone replacement therapy: the postmenopausal estrogen/progestin intervention (PEPI) trial," *J. Women's Health Gend Based Med* 1999; 8(9):1167–1172.

402. Tallova, J., et al., "Changes of plasma total homocysteine levels during the menstrual cycle," *Eur J. Clin Invest* 1999; 29(12):1041–1044.

403. Stoney, C., et al., "Plasma homocysteine levels increase in women during psychological stress," *Life Sci* 1999; 64(25):2359–2365.

404. Drouva, S., et al., "Estradiol activates methylating enzyme(s) involved in the conversion of phosphatidylcholine in rat pituitary membranes," *Endocrinol* 1986; 119(6):2611–2622.

405. Sinatra, S., *Optimum Health*, Gatlinburg, TN:The Lincoln-Bradley Publishing Group, 1996; p. 164.

406. Ellison, P., .et al., "Measurements of salivary progesterone," *Annals of the New York Academy of Science* 1993; 694:161–76.

407. Vining, R., et al., "The measurements of hormones in saliva: possibility and pitfalls," *J. of Steroid Biochem* 1987; 27:81–94.

408. Vining R., et al., "Hormones in saliva: mode of entry and consequent implications for clinical interpretation," *Clinical Chemistry* 1983; 29(10):1752–1756.

409. Henderson, V., et al., "The epidemiology of estrogen replacement therapy and Alzheimer's disease," *Neurology* 1997; 48:S27–S35.

410. Sherman, B., et al., "Estrogen use and verbal memory in healthy postmenopausal women," *Obstet and Gynecol* 1994; 83(6):979–83.

411. Ibid., Tang, p. 429–32.

412. Vliet, E., et al., "New insights on hormones and mood," *Menopause Management* 1993; June/July:140–146.

413. Prior, J., et al., "Progesterone as a bone-tropic hormone," *Endocrine Reviews* 1990; 11:386–98.

414. Yang, C., et al., "Efficacy and safety of estriol replacement therapy for climacteric women," *Am J. of Obstet Gynecol* 1995; 173:670–671.

415. Bender, S., *The Power of Perimenopause.* 1998; New York: Harmony Books, p. 168.

416. Ahlgrimm, M., *The HRT Solution.* 1999; New York:Avery Publishing, p. 22.

417. Ibid., Ahligrimm, p. 28.

418. Ibid., Ahligrimm, p. 35.

419. Ibid., Ahligrimm, p. 43.

420. Ibid., Ahligrimm, p. 55.

421. Ibid., Ahligrimm, p. 55.

422. Ibid., Ahligrimm, p. 55.

423. Ibid., Ahligrimm, p. 98.

424. Ibid., Ahligrimm, p. 113.

425. Ibid., Ahligrimm, p. 113.

426. Brownstein, D., *Overcoming Thyroid Disorders.* West Bloomfield, MI: Medical Alternatives Press, 2002, p. 8.

427. Ibid., Brownstein, p. 27.

428. Ibid., Brownstein, p. 37.

429. Horst, C., et al., "Rapid stimulation of hepatic oxygen consumption by 3,5-di-iodo-1-thyrooninne," *Biochem J.* 1989; 261:945–950.

430. Vunevicious., B., et al., "Effects of thyroxine as compared with thyroxine plus triiodothyronine in patients with hypothyroidism," *NEJM* 1999; 340:424–429.

431. Fed Regester August 14, 1997; 62(157).

432. Ibid., Brownstein, *Overcoming Thyroid Disorders*, p. 51.

433. Ibid., Brownstein, p. 113.

434. Ibid., Brownstein, p. 136.

435. Barrett-Conner, E., et al., "A prospective study of dehydroepiandrosterone sulfate, mortality and cardiovascular disease," *NEJM* 1986; 37(9); 1035.

436. Ibid., Brownstein, *Overcoming Thyroid Disorders*, p. 140.

437. Gordon, G., et al., "Reduction of atherosclerosis by administration of dehydroepiandrosterone. A study of the hypercholesterolemic New Zealand white rabbit with aortic internal injury," *J. Clin Invest* 1988; 82:712.

438. Schairer, C., et al., "Menopausal estrogen and estrogen-progestin replacement therapy's breast cancer risk," *JAMA* 2000; 283:485–491.

439. Pansini, F., "Effect of the hormonal contraception on serum reverse triiodothyronine levels," *Gynecol Obstet Invest* 1987; 23:133.

440. Tagawa, N., et al., "Serum dehydroepiandrosterone, dehydroepiandrosterone sulfate, and pregnenolone sulfate concentrations in patients with hyperthyroidism and hypothyroidism," *Clinical Chem* 2000; 46:523–528.

441. Nishida, M., et al., "Direct evidence for the presence of methylmercury bound in the thyroid and other organs obtained from mice give methylmercury; differentiation of free and bound methylmercuries in biological materials determined by volatility of methylmercury," *Chem Pharm Bull* 1990; 38(5):1412–3.

442. Haggins, C. et al., "The effect of flaxseed and wheat bran consumption on urinary estrogen metabolites in premenopausal woman," *Cancer Epidemiology Biomarkers and Prevention* 2000; 9:719–725.

443. Osborn, M., et al., "Omega 3 fatty acids: modulation of estrogen metabolism and potential for breast cancer prevention," *Cancer Invest* 1988; 8:629–631.

444. Boggs, D., et al., "Effects of a very low fat, high fiber diet on serum hormones and menstrual function, implications for breast cancer prevention," *Cancer* 1995; 76:2491–2496.

445. Collins, J., *What's Your Menopause Type*. Roseville, CA:Prima Health, 2000.

446. Ibid., Bradlow, *Environ Health Prospect* p. 147–150.

447. Ibid., Bradlow, p. 147–150.

448. Bradlow, H., et al., "16-alpha-hydroxylation of estradiol: a possible risk marker for breast cancer," *Ann NY Acad Sci* 1986; 464:138–51.

449. Ibid., Muti, p. 635–40.

450. Ibid., Fishman, p. 1077–81.

451. Ibid., Melilahn, p. 1250–1255.

452. Lahita, R., et al., "Abnormal estrogen and androgen metabolism in the human with systemic lupus erythematosus," *Am J. Kidney Dis* 1982; 2(1suppl1):206–11.

453. Lahita, R., et al., "Determination of 16-alpha-hydroxyestrone by radioimmunoassay in systemic lupus erythematosus," *Arthritis Rheum* 1985; 28(10):1122–7.

454. Dupont, E., et al., "Prognostic value of altered estrogen metabolism in breast cancer patients on premarin. Poster session abstract presented at the 37th American Society of Clinical Oncology Meeting 2001.

455. Dupont, E., et al., "The prognostic value of altered estrogen metabolism in breast cancer," *Ann Surg Oncol* 2000; 7(1)suppl.

456. Fowke, J., et al., "Macronutrient intake and estrogen metabolism in healthy postmenopausal women," *Breast Cancer Res Treat* 2001; 65(1):1–10.

457. Haggans, C., et al., "The effect of flaxseed and wheat bran consumption on urinary estrogen metabolites in premenopausal women," *Cancer Epidemiol Biomarkers Prev* 2000; 9(7):719–725.

458. Haggans, C., et al., "Effect of flaxseed consumption on urinary estrogen metabolites in postmenopausal women," *Nutr Cancer* 1999; 33(2):188–95.

459. Ibid., Fowke, 779.

460. Bradlow, H., et al., "Effects of pesticides on the ratio of 16-alpha/2hydroxyestrone: a biologic marker of breast cancer risk," *Environ Health Perspect* 1995; 103(suppl 7):147–50.

461. Lu, L., et al., "Increased urinary excretion of 2-hydroxyestrone but not 16-alpha-hydroxyestrone in premenopausal women during a soy diet containing isoflavones," *Cancer Res* 2000; 60(5):1299–305.

462. Ibid., Vliet, p. 149.

463. Lewis, A., *Melatonin and the Biological Clock*. New Canann, Connecticut: Keats Publishing, 1996.

464. Ibid., Vliet, p. 150.

465. Ibid., Vliet, p. 150.

466. Ibid., Vliet, p. 154.

467. Ibid., Vliet, p. 157.

468. Ibid., Vliet, p. 202.

469. Ibid., Vliet, p. 203.

470. Ibid., Vliet, p. 217.

471. Ibid., Vliet, p. 218.

472. Ibid., Vliet, p. 224.

473. Ibid., Vliet, p. 302.

474. Ibid., Vliet, p. 242.

475. Ibid., Vliet, p. 227.

476. Ibid., Vliet, p. 231.

477. Springer-Verlag, S., *Testosterone: Action, Deficiency, Substitution.* Berlin, 1998, p. 299.

478. Hofman, T., et al., "Steroid hormones in saliva," *Diagnostic Endocrinol Met* 1998; 16(9):265–273.

479. Mandel, I., et al., "The diagnostic use of saliva," *J. Oral Pathol Med* 1990; 19:119–125.

480. Riad-Fahney, L., et al., "Steroids in saliva for assessing endocrine function," *Endocr Rev* 1982; 3(4):367–95.

481. Brineat, M., et al., "Long-tern effects of the menopause and sex hormones on skin thickness," *Br J. Obstet Gynaecol* 1985; 92(3):256–259.

482. Jacobs, D., et al., "Cognitive function in nondeminated older women who took estrogen after menopause," *Neurology* 1998; 50(2):368–373.

483. Sherwin, B., et al., "Estrogen effects on cognition in menopausal women," *Neurology* 1997: 48(suppl 7):S21–S26.

484. Kampen, D., et al., "Estrogen use and verbal memory in healthy post-menopausal women" *Obstet Gynecol* 1994; 83(6):979–983.

485. Rice, M., et al., "Estrogen replacement therapy and cognitive function in postmenopausal women without dementia," *Am J. Med* 1997; 103(3A):26S–35S.

486. Anderson, V., et al., "Estrogen, cognition and woman's risk of Alzheimer's disease," *Am J. Med* 1997; 103(3A):11S–18S.

487. Heikkinen, A., et al., "Post-menopausal hormone replacement therapy and autoantibodies against oxidized LDL," *Maturitas* 1998; 29(2):155–161.

488. Haines, C., et al., "An examination of the effect of combined cyclical hormone replacement therapy on lipoprotein (a) and other lipoproteins," *Atheroscleorosis* 1996; 119(2):215–222.

489. Espeland, E., et al., "Effect of postmenopausal hormone replacement therapy on lipoprotein (a) concentration: PEPI Investigators Postmenopausal Estrogen/Progestin Interven-tions," *Circulation* 1998; 97(10):979–986.

490. Wouters, M., et al., "Plasma homocysteine and menopausal statues," *Eur J. Clin Invest* 1995; 25(11):801–805.

491. Nasr, A., et al., "Estrogen replacement therapy and cardio-vascular protection: lipid mechanisms are the tip of an iceberg," *Gynecol Endocrinol* 1998; 12(1):43–59.

492. Sudhir, L., et al., "Estrogen supplementation decreases norepinephrine-induced vasoconstriction and total body norepinephrine spillover in perimenopausal women," *Hypertension* 1997; 30(6):1538–1543.

493. Sacks, F, et al., "Sex hormones, lipoproteins, and vascular reactivity," *Curr Opin Lipodol* 1995; 6(3):161–166.

494. Ibid., Collins, p. 67.

495. Ibid., Collins, p. 69.

496. Khastigir, G., et al., "Hysterectomy, ovarian failure and depression," *Menopause* 1996; 5(2):113–122.

497. Persky, H., et al., "Plasma testosterone level and sexual behavior of couples," *Arch Sex Behav* 1978; 7(3):157–173.

498. Brincat, M., et al., "Sex hormones and skin collagen content in postmenopausal woman," *Br Med J.* 1983; 287(6402):1337–1338.

499. Davis, S., et al., "Use of androgens in postmenopausal women," *Curr Opin Obstet Gynecol* 1997; 9(3):177–180.

500. Surrel, P., et al., "Cardiovascular aspects of androgens in women," *Semin Repro Endocrinol* 1998; 16(2):121–128.

501. Bruning, P., et al., "Insulin resistance and breast cancer risk," *Int J. Cancer* 1992; 52(4):511–516.

502. Stroll, B., et al., "Essential fatty acids, insulin resistance and breast cancer risk," *Nutr Cancer* 1998; 31(1):72–77.

503. Colacurci, N., et al., "Effects of hormone replacement therapy on glucose metabolism," *Panminerva Med* 1998; 40(1):18–21.

504. Anderson, B., et al., "Estrogen replacement therapy decreases hyperandrogenicity and improves glucose homeostasis: Plasma lipids in postmenopausal women with NIDDM," *J. Clinc Endocrin* 1997; 82(2):638–643.

505. Khaw, K., et al., "Fasting plasma glucose levels and endogenous androgens in non-diabetic postmenopausal women," *Clin Sci* 1991; 80(3):199–203.

506. Haffner, S., et al., "Endogenous sex hormones: impact on lipids, lipoproteins, and insulin," *Am J. Med* 1995; 98(1A):40S–47S.

507. Ibid., Collins, p. 79.

508. Ibid., Collins, p. 88.

509. Ibid., Collins, p. 171.

510. Schmidt, J., et al., Other anti-androgens," *Dermatology* 1998; 196(1):153–157.

511. Ibid., Collins, p. 174.

512. Ibid., Collins, p. 181.

513. Beattie, J., et al., "The influence of a low boron diet and boron supplementation on bone, major mineral and sex steroid metabo-lism in post-menopausal women," *Br J. Nutrition* 1993; 49(3):871–884.

514. Naghii, M., et al., "The role of boron in nutrition and metabo-lism," *Prog Food Nutr Sci* 1993; 17(4):331–349.

515. Hunt, C., et al., "Dietary boron modifies the effects of vitamin D3 nutrition on indices of energy substrate utilization and mineral metabolism in the chick," *J. Bone Miner Res* 1994; 9(2):171–182.

516. Ibid., Collins, p. 182.

517. Mathias, S., et al., "Modulation of adrenal cell function by cadmium salts. 4 Ca(2+)-dependent sites affected by Cd C12 during basal and ACTH-stimulated steroid synthesis," *Cell Biol Toxicol* 1998; 14(3):225–236.

518. Matsuki, M., et al., "Effects of calcium channel blockers on steroidogenesis stimulated by ACTH and cAMP in isolated rat adrenal cells," *Horm Metab Res* 1996; 28(8):374–376.

519. Scheen, A., et al., "Perspective in the treatment of insulin resistance," *Hum Reprod* 1997; 12(suppl 1):63–71.

520. Barnes, M., et al., "The effects of vitamin E deficiency on some enzymes of steroid hormone biosynthesis," *Int J. Vitamin Nut Res* 1975; 45(4):396–403.

521. Ibid., Collins, p. 189.

522. Ibid., Collins, p. 189.

523. Reddy, R., et al., "Effects of vanadyl sulphate on ornithine decarboxylase and progesterone levels in the ovary of rat," *Biochem Int* 1989; 18(2):467–474.

524. Lindeman, R., "Trace minerals: hormonal and metabolic interrelationships," *Principles, Practice of Endocrinolgy and Metabolism.* Philadelphia: J.B. Lippincott, 1995.

525. Ibid., Collins, p. 192.

526. Omura, T., et al., "Gene regulation of steroidogenesis," *J. Steroid Biochem Mol Biol* 1995; 53(1–6):19–25.

527. Ibid., Collins, p. 192.

528. Kamada, H., et al., "Effect of selenium on cultured bovine luteal cells," *Anim Reprod Sci* 1997; 46(3–4):203–211.

529. Wolf, C., et al., "Effect of natural oestrogens on tryptophan metabolism: evidence of interference of oestrogens with kyneureninase," *Scand J. Clin Lab Invest* 1980; 40(1):15–22.

530. Musicki, B., "Endocrine regulation of ascorbic acid transport and secretion in luteal cells," *Bio Reprod* 1996; 54(2):399–406.

531. Ibid., Collins, p. 204.

532. Aten, R., et al., "Ovarian vitamin E accumulation: evidence for a role of lipoproteins," *Endocrinology* 1994; 135(2):533–539.

533. Minshall, R., et al., "Ovarian steroid protection against coronary artery hyperreactivity in rhesus monkeys," *J. Clin Endocrinol Metab* 1998; 83(2):649–659.

534. Ibid., Collins, p. 277.

535. Ibid., Collins, p. 285.

536. van der Linden, M., et al., "The effect of estriol on the cytology of urethra and vagina in post-menopausal women with genito-urinary symptoms," *Eur J. Obstet Gynecol Reprod Biol* 1993; 51(1):29–33.

537. Ibid., Collins, p. 291.

538. McAuley, J., et al. "Oral administration of micronized progesterone; a review and more experience," *Pharmacotherapy* 1996; 16(3):453–457.

539. Miodrg, A., et al., "Sex hormones and the female urinary tract," *Drugs* 1988; 36(4):491–504.

540. Sarrel, P., et al., "Cardiovascular aspects of androgens in women," *Semin Reprod Endocrinol* 1998; 16(2):121–128.

541. Sarrel, P., et al., "Vasodilator effects of estrogen are not diminished by androgen in postmenopausal women," *Fertil Steril* 1997; 68(6): 1125–1127.

542. Sinatra, S., *Heart Sense for Women.* Washington D.C.: LifeLine Press, 2000, p. 108.

543. Ibid., Sinatra, p. 205.

544. Ibid., Sinatra, p. 205.

545. Ibid., Sinatra, p. 206.

546. Ibid., Sinatra, p. 207.

547. Chadhurz, N., et al., "Antioxidant and pro-oxidant actions of estrogens: potential physiological and clinical implications," *Seminars in Reproductive Endocrin* 1998; 16(4):309–314.

548. Ibid., Sinatra, p. 208.

549. Ibid., Sinatra, p. 208.

550. Ibid., Sinatra, p. 210.

551. Ibid., Sinatra, p. 211.

552. Ibid., Sinatra, p. 211.

553. Ibid., Sinatra, p. 212.

554. Ibid., Sinatra, p. 212.

555. Ibid., Sinatra, p. 212.

556. Ibid., Sinatra, p. 214.

557. Ibid., Sinatra, p. 216.

558. Ibid., Sinatra, p. 216.

559. Ibid., Sinatra, p. 217.

560. Ibid., Sinatra, p. 218.

561. Ibid., Sinatra, p. 218.

562. Ibid., Sinatra, p. 219.

563. Ibid., Sinatra, p. 219.

564. Ibid., Sinatra, p. 219.

565. Ibid., Sinatra, p. 53.

566. Ibid., Sinatra, p. 53.

567. Ibid., Sinatra, p. 53.

568. Ibid., Sinatra, p. 54.

569. Ibid., Sinatra, p. 54.

570. Ibid., Sinatra, p. 55.

571. Ibid., Sinatra, p. 55.

572. Ibid., Sinatra, p. 55.

573. Ibid., Sinatra, p. 62.

574. Ibid., Sinatra, p. 63.

575. Ibid., Sinatra, p. 63.

576. Ibid., Sinatra, p. 64.

577. Ibid., Sinatra, p. 66.

578. Ibid., Sinatra, p. 66.

579. Ibid., Sinatra, p. 68.

580. Ibid., Sinatra, p. 69.

581. Sherwin, B., et al., "Estrogenic effects on memory in women," *Am NY Acad Sci* 1994; 743:213–230, 230–31.

582. Ibid., Sinatra, Optimum Health, p. 164.

583. The Importance of Detoxification, 2002; Advanced Nutritional Publications, Inc.

584. Ibid., *The Importance of Detoxification*.

585. Ibid., *The Importance of Detoxification*.

586. Ibid., *The Importance of Detoxification*.

587. Lazarou, J., et al., "Incidence of adverse drug reaction in hospitalized patients," *JAMA* 1998; 279(15):1200–1205.

588. Great Smokies Diagnostic Laboratory (See appendix).

589. Great Smokies Diagnostic Laboratory (See appendix).

590. Holtzman, N., "Will genetics revolutionize medicine," *NEJM* 2000; 343(2):78–85.

591. Thompson, N., et al., "Exisulind induction of apoptosis involves guanosine 3',5'-cyclic monophosphate phosphodiesterase inhibitor, protein kinase activation and attenuated B-catenin," *Cancer Res* 2000; 60:3338–3342.

592. Phillips, K., et al., "Potential role of pharmacogenomics in reducing adverse drugs reactions," *JAMA* 2001; 268(18):2270–2279.

593. Goodman & Gilman, *Pharmacological Basis of Therapeutics*, 1996; New York: McGraw-Hill.

594. Foss-Morgan, R., *Hormone Replacement Therapy*. Haddonfield, New Jersey: AntiAging and Longevity Medical Center of Haddonfield, 2000.

595. Germano, R., The Osteoporosis Solution. New York:Kensington Publishing Corp., 1999, p. 102.

596. Ibid., Germano, p. 102.

597. Ibid., Germano, p. 103.

598. Ibid., Germano, p. 99.

599. Ibid., Germano, p. 101.

600. Ibid., Nachtigall, p. 154.

601. Crook, T., *The Memory Cure.* New York:Pocket Books, 1998, p. 159.

602. Ibid., Crook, p. 234.

603. Colgan, M., *The New Nutrition.* Vancover:Apple Publishing, 1995, p. 64.

604. Ibid., Colgan, p. 63.

605. Ibid., Colgan, p. 102–103.

606. Ibid., Colgan, p. 101.

607. Ibid., Colgan, p. 104.

608. Ibid., Laux, p. 48–149.

609. Ibid., Germano, p. 91.

610. Gittleman, A. *Super Nutrition For Menopause.* New York:Avery Publishing, 1998, p. 52–53.

611. Ibid., Gittleman, p. 79.

612. Ibid., Germano, p. 104.

613. Ibid., Lieberman, p. 85.

614. Ibid., Gittleman, p. 61.

615. Ibid., Lieberman, p. 165.

616. Ibid., Germano, p. 42.

617. Ibid., Laux, p. 75–76.

618. Bland, J., "Nutritional endocrinology: the estrogen-testosterone-progesterone connection to hypothalamus, pituitary, adrenal, thyroid and endocrine pancreas function," *Breakthrough Approaches For Improving Adrenal and Thyroid Function.* Gig Harbor:Metagenics, Inc., 2002, p.131–132.

619. Chen, Y., et al., "The equine estrogen metabolite 4-hydroxyequilenin cause DNS single-strand breaks and oxidation of DNA bases in vitro," *Chem Res Toxicol* 1998; 11:1105–111.

620. Yagi, E., et al., "The ability of four catechol estrogens of 17 B-estradiol and estrone to induce DNA adducts in Syrian hamster embryo fibroblasts," *Carcinogenesis* 2001; 22 (9):1505–1510.

621. Pish, E., et al., "Evidence that a metabolite of equine estrogens 4-hydroxy equilenin, induces cellular transformation in vitro," *Chem Res Toxicol* 2001; 14:82–90.

622. Meng, Q., et al., "Inhibitory effects of indole-3-carbinol on invasion and migration in human breast cancer cells," *Breast Cancer Res Treatment* 2000; 63:147–152.

623. Ibid., Michnovicz, *J. Natl Cancer Inst.*, p. 718–723.

624. Ford, E., et al., "Homocysteine and cardiovascular disease: a systemic review of the evidence with special emphasis on case-control studies and nested case-control studies," *Int J. Epidemiol* 2002; 31(1):59–70.

625. Clarke, R, et al., "Underestimation of the importance of homocysteine as a risk factor for cardiovascular disease in epidemiological studies," *J. Cardiovasc Risk* 2001; 8(6):363–9.

626. Rost, N, et al., "Plasma concentration of C-reactive protein and risk of ischemic stroke and transient ischemic attack: the Framingham study," *Stroke* 2001; 32(11):2575–9.

627. Ridker, P., et al., "Novel risk factors for systemic atherosclerosis: a comparison of C-reactive protein, fibrinogen, homocysteine, lipoprotein (a) and standard cholesterol screening as predictors of peripheral arterial disease," *JAMA* 2001; 285(19):2481–5.

628. Ibid., Ridker, p. 2481–5.

629. Matsumoto, Y., et al., "High level of lipoprotein (a) is a strong predictor for progression of coronary artery disease," *J. Atharoscler Thromb* 1998; 5(2):47–53.

630. <http://www.dr.sinatra.com/> Dec. 19, 2001.

631. Ibid., dr.sinatra.com, Dec. 19, 2001.

632. Schmidt, J., et al., "Treatment of skin aging with topical estrogens," *International Journal of Pharmaceutical Compounding* 1998; 2(4):270–275.

633. Jialal, I., et al., "Inflammation and atherosclerosis: the value of the high-sensitivity c-reactive protein assay as a risk marker," *Am J Clin Pathol* 2001; 116 Suppl:S108–15.

634. Madsen, T., et al., "C-reactive protein, dietary n-3 fatty acids, and the extent of coronary artery disease," *Am J Cardiol* 2001; 88(10):1139–42.

635. Ford, E., et al., "Does exercise reduce inflammation? Physical activity and c-reactive protein among U.S. adults," *Epidemiology* 2002; 13(5):561–8.

636. Zandi, P., et al., "Hormone replacement therapy and incidence of Alzheimer disease in older women," *JAMA* 2002; 288(17):2123–2129.

637. Kanaya, A., et al., "Glycemic effects of postmenopausal hormone therapy: the heart and estrogen/progestin replacement study," *Ann Intern Med* 2003; 138(1):1–9.

Give the Gift of
HRT: The Answers
to Your Friends and Colleagues

CHECK YOUR LEADING BOOKSTORE OR ORDER HERE

❑ **YES**, I want _____ copies of *HRT* at $17.95 each, plus $4.95 shipping per book (Michigan residents please add $1.08 sales tax per book). Canadian orders must be accompanied by a postal money order in U.S. funds. Allow 15 days for delivery.

❑ **YES**, I am interested in having Dr. Pamela Smith speak or give a seminar to my company, association, school, or organization. Please send information.

My check or money order for $_____ is enclosed.

Please charge my ❑ Visa ❑ MasterCard ❑ Discover ❑ American Express

Name _____

Organization _____

Address _____

City/State/Zip _____

Phone_____ E-mail _____

Card # _____

Exp. Date_____ Signature _____

Please make your check payable and return to:
Healthy Living Books, Inc.
575 S. Long Lake Road • Traverse City, MI 49684

Call or fax your credit card order to: 1-231-943-4577
or contact:
The Center For Healthy Living and Longevity
www.healthliving.meta-ehealth.com